HOW TO PREPARE
FOR THE
STEP 1 MEDICAL EXAM

Second Edition

NOTICE

Medicine is an ever-changing science. As new research and clinical experience broaden our knowledge, changes in treatment and drug therapy are required. The authors and the publisher of this work have checked with sources believed to be reliable in their efforts to provide information that is complete and generally in accord with the standards accepted at the time of publication. However, in view of the possibility of human error or changes in medical sciences, neither the authors, nor the publisher, nor any other party who has been involved in the preparation or publication of this work warrants that the information contained herein is in every respect accurate or complete and they are not responsible for any errors or omissions or for the results obtained from use of such information. Readers are encouraged to confirm the information contained herein with other sources. For example and in particular, readers are advised to check the product information sheet included in the package of each drug they plan to administer to be certain that the information contained in this book is accurate and that changes have not been made in the recommended dose or in the contraindications for administration. This recommendation is of particular importance in connection with new or infrequently use drugs.

A PreTest® Publication

HOW TO PREPARE FOR THE STEP 1 MEDICAL EXAM

Second Edition

John R. Thornborough, Ph.D.
Mount Sinai School of Medicine
of The City University of New York

Hilary J. Schmidt, Ph.D.
State University of New York
Health Science Center at Brooklyn

McGraw-Hill, Inc.
Health Professions Division

New York   St. Louis   San Francisco   Auckland
Bogotá   Caracas   Lisbon   London   Madrid
Mexico   Milan   Montreal   New Delhi   Paris
San Juan   Singapore   Sydney   Tokyo   Toronto

HOW TO PREPARE FOR THE STEP 1 MEDICAL EXAM
SECOND EDITION

Figures for question 25 of Behavior Test II from Pattishall, *Behavioral Sciences: PreTest® Self-Assessment and Review*, 5/e, New York: McGraw-Hill, 1991; with permission. Figures for questions 4 and 21 of Biochemistry Test II from Chlapowski, *Biochemistry: PreTest® Self-Assessment and Review*, 6/e, New York: McGraw-Hill, 1991; with permission. Figures for questions 11, 12, 17, and 19 of Microbiology Test II from Tilton and Buchanan, *Microbiology: PreTest® Self-Assessment and Review*, 6/e, New York: McGraw-Hill, 1991; with permission. Figures for questions 4, 8, and 24 of Pathology Test I, and questions 4, 6, 7, 18, 20, and 21 of Pathology Test II from Clements, *Pathology: PreTest® Self-Assessment and Review*, 6/e, New York: McGraw-Hill, 1991; with permission. Figures for questions 2, 11-13, and 14 of Physiology Test I, and questions 1, 3, 7, 13, 15, and 17 of Physiology Test II from Mulligan, *Physiology: PreTest® Self-Assessment and Review*, 6/e, New York: McGraw-Hill, 1991; with permission.

1 2 3 4 5 6 7 8 9 0 DOCDOC 9 9 8 7 6 5 4 3

ISBN 0-07-064522-1

This book was set in Times Roman by ILOC, Inc.
The editor was Gail Gavert.
The production supervisors were Clara B. Stanley and Gyl Favours.
R.R. Donnelley & Sons was printer and binder.

Library of Congress Cataloging-in-Publication

Thornborough, John R.
    How to prepare for the step 1 medical exam/ John R. Thornborough, Hilary J. Schmidt.-- 2nd ed.
        p.   cm.
    Rev. ed. of: How to prepare for the National Medical Board examination comprehensive part I. c1991.
        ISBN 0-07-064522-1 :
        1. Medicine--Examinations, questions, etc. 2. Medical sciences--Examinations, questions, etc. 3. National Board of Medical Examiners--Examinations--Study guides. I. Schmidt, Hilary J. II. Thornborough, John R. How to prepare for the National Medical Board examination comprehensive part I. III. Title..
        [DNLM: 1. Educational Measurement. 2. Medicine--examination questions. W 18 T497h]
    R834.5.T47 1993
    610'.76--dc20
    DNLM/DLC
    for Library of Congress   92-48780
                                                                              CIP

CONTENTS

PREFACE

This book is about how to prepare for and pass your licensure examination. It has been extensively revised from the first edition. It explains how to get organized, how to choose study materials, how to decide what to study, how much time to spend, how to study effectively, how to study efficiently, how to test yourself, and how to take the board examination. Also, in this edition we have included several practice examinations for your use. Be sure to take advantage of them.

All this how-to information comes from many years of experience working with many different medical students, both those who have failed and those who have passed the boards. Thus, the review program presented in this book is based not only on cognitive psychology theory but also on our successful application of this program with a large number of students.

You do not have time for long, complex books about how to study, so we put the important points in boxes and **bold type**, and we present what you need to know in a clear, straightforward manner. Thus, this concise book is quick and easy to read.

If you use all the hints, tips, ideas, and plans presented here, you will undertake the most efficient and effective review possible. Realistically, however, you probably will adopt some recommendations more than others. If you do this, be sure that you select wisely and do not compromise your overall goals.

Whatever you do, be sure to **read Chapter 7 to design your review plan and to implement it**. We cannot stress enough that the most important thing you can do to ensure that you review efficiently and effectively and, therefore, do well on the board examination is to plan a review program and schedule your time before the exam.

Good luck with your studies and with the exam. This book should help you with both.

Chapter 1

Introduction to the United States Medical Licensing Examination

This chapter describes the examination and its design, content, question types, and rules.

OVERVIEW The United States Medical Licensing Examination Step 1 (USMLE) is the first of three examinations leading to licensing of a physician. The purpose of Step 1 is to determine if you know and can use fundamental concepts of the basic medical sciences. You should **not** think of it as merely a collection of seven examinations, one in each of the seven basic sciences; rather, it is a comprehensive test of all the basic biomedical sciences. The designers of this examination have tried to integrate their questions across all these sciences. It emphasizes the concepts that serve as a basis for clinical medicine and disease prevention and also requires that you recall certain factual information. Thus, in reviewing for this examination, you should attempt to integrate material that may have been presented to you in a course-by-course structure as well as to commit basic "facts" to memory. Suggestions in subsequent chapters in this book will help you to plan and organize such a conceptually integrative, factual review.

FORMAT The examination consists of approximately 800 multiple-choice questions presented in four books over the course of two days. The total examination time is 12 hours. Thus, you will have between 50 seconds and 1 minute to answer each question . More time may be spent on some items and less on others, but your total testing time will be fixed at 3 hours for each of the four books of approximately 200 questions.

QUESTION TYPES The examination consists of two basic types of questions: the single best answer question and matching questions (headings). Following are examples of each type:

One Best Answer

All of the following are known to cause splenomegaly EXCEPT
    A. sickle cell disease
    B. Hodgkin's disease
    C. chronic lymphocytic leukemia (CLL)
    D. hairy cell leukemia
    E. polycythemia vera

(5 options A to E)

(See **Pathology: PreTest® Self-Assessment and Review**, 6th ed. p. 70 for a discussion of this question.)

Matching Sets

For each of the preparations below, choose the virus or disease to which it is most closely related.
    A. Hepatitis A
    B. Influenza A
    C. Measles
    D. Herpes simplex
    E. Hepatitis B
(4 to 26 response options per question)
1. Acylovir
2. Pooled serum immune globulin
3. Killed virus vaccine

(See **Microbiology: PreTest® Self-Assessment and Review**, 6th ed. p. 16, for a discussion of these questions.)

THE DIMENSIONS OF STEP 1.

		SYSTEMS (DIMENSION 1.)	
		General Principles (40 - 50%) e.g., homeostasis	Individual OrganSystems (50 - 60%) e.g., cardiovascular
PROCESS (DIMENSION 2)	Normal Processes (45 - 55%)	ORGANIZATIONAL LEVEL (DIMENSION 3) 15-25% - Person (e.g., society, family, individual) 50-60% - Organ/tissue Cell/subcellular Molecular 15-25% - Nonhuman organism Exogenous substance	ORGANIZATIONAL LEVEL (DIMENSION 3) 15-25% - Person (e.g., society, family, individual) 50-60% - Organ/tissue Cell/subcellular Molecular 15-25% - Nonhuman organism Exogenous substance
	Abnormal Processes (45 - 55%)	ORGANIZATIONAL LEVEL (DIMENSION 3) 15-25% - Person (e.g., society, family, individual) 50-60% - Organ/tissue Cell/subcellular Molecular 15-25% - Nonhuman organism Exogenous substance	ORGANIZATIONAL LEVEL (DIMENSION 3) 15-25% - Person (e.g., society, family, individual) 50-60% - Organ/tissue Cell/subcellular Molecular 15-25% - Nonhuman organism Exogenous substance

CONTENT The content of the examination is drawn from the seven basic science subjects: anatomy, behavioral science, biochemistry, microbiology, pathology, pharmacology, and physiology. Questions are written by faculty members from Canadian and U.S. medical schools serving on individual subject committees and also on multidisciplinary committees. The examination is based on a content outline organized in three dimensions (see the diagram on page 3). You should carefully study the complete content outline for the examination found in **Step 1 General Instructions, Content Outline and Sample Items**, published each year by the Federation of State Medical Boards of the U.S., Inc. and the National Board of Medical Examiners.

RULES You will not be permitted to take any books, notes, calculators, paging devices, recording devices of any kind, radios, or any other electronic devices, including wrist watches with memories, into the testing room with you. Talking to other examinees during the test is not permitted. If you must, you may leave the testing room temporarily but only in the presence of an escort. If you do leave, however, you will **not** receive any extra time to compensate for your absence from the test.

DATES Step 1 is offered twice a year, in June and in September. Students generally sit for this test at the end of their second year of medical school. You will register for a particular administration approximately six months in advance of its scheduled date. To do so, you must be sponsored by your medical school.

SCORES You must complete all four books of the examination in order to receive a score. Each question is worth one point when answered correctly and there is no scoring penalty for incorrect answers or omissions. Passing is determined on the basis of a total score. According to the National Board of Medical Examiners, in June 1990 58% was the minimum passing score, and in 1991 it was 53%. This requirement will probably not change significantly in the future. Scores are usually mailed to examinees about one month after the administration of the examination.

Chapter 2

Learning, Forgetting, and Memory Savings

This chapter describes some principles of learning and memory (and forgetting).

INTRODUCTION Learning about the mechanisms of memory and forgetting is important since it should help you to...

— identify areas which will require more intensive review than others.

— learn about review methods that should optimize gains.

— design an optimal study plan for USMLE.

Human memory is governed by rules, one of which is that we forget much of what we learn. Forgetting is a fact of life and, unfortunately, immediately after learning new information (and being tested on it), you can expect to start forgetting it. This means that the subjects you studied during your first year in medical school and knew quite well at the time may have suffered from memory loss. Even your most recently learned information is undergoing forgetting. Fortunately, you can learn to minimize this normal forgetting process. Indeed, your future career as a physician depends upon your ability to recall and use the large amount of information that you learn in medical school. The amount of information that you will be able to recall and use on the USMLE will be related to...

MEMORY RECOMMENDATIONS Below is a listing of certain facts and recommendations related to memory that should be considered when deciding what, when, and how to review for the National Board examination:

1. **Familiarity should not be equated with knowing.** One of the greatest hazards when reviewing for the board examination is assuming that being familiar with information indicates an adequate level of knowledge. Almost everything you review will seem familiar, since most of it has been learned before. But familiarity does not mean that you will be able to recall the information during a testing situation or, even if you recall it, be able to use the information to solve problems. To illustrate this, consider an American penny. Everyone "knows" what a penny looks like. After all, each of us has seen thousands of pennies. <u>But familiarity with the penny does not guarantee that you will be able to recognize the penny.</u>   Look at the pennies illustrated below:

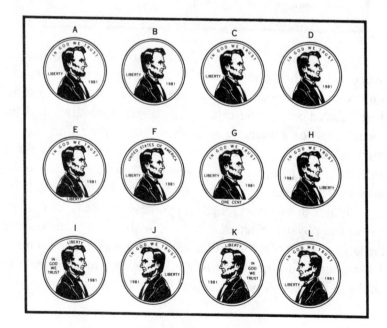

Which one is an accurate drawing of the U.S. penny? Circle the one you think is correct and then take out a real penny and compare. How did you do?[1]

WHEN REVIEWING FOR USMLE

— **ESSAY** Study as if for an essay examination as opposed to a multiple-choice examination. This forces you to organize and summarize your knowledge into coherent bodies of information as opposed to learning lists of facts. Research shows that preparing for an essay examination leads to significantly better performance on multiple-choice examinations than does preparing for a multiple-choice examination itself.

— **SELF-TEST** As you review, always test whether or not you can recall the information that is presented in your source. Use practice questions to evaluate your knowledge on a regular basis.

— **ANTICIPATE** As you study, try to anticipate what information will be included in each section of your review book.

— **HIGHLIGHT** As you review, identify (e.g., highlight) information that you did not remember, did not know, or are having difficulty understanding.

---

[1] Nickerson, R.S. & Adams, M.J. (1979). Long-term memory for a common object. Cognitive Psychology 11, 287-307.

2. **Understanding increases memory retention and recall** and leads to better problem solving. Subjects or topics that you did not understand well as you learned them will be subject to more forgetting than subjects you did understand well. Facts that were memorized by rote (e.g., formulas) without understanding may have been forgotten altogether. Topics that were well understood and not memorized by rote will require less time to review.

3. **Active learning greatly increases subsequent recall.** Summarizing and reorganizing information by making charts, drawing pictures or diagrams, and mentally visualizing are all active learning strategies that promote long-term retention. If you did not use these strategies when learning material the first time, you will need more time to review later.

If you did make summaries, charts, and other forms of condensed notes while you were taking your courses, you will not only more easily recall that information but also find that these materials constitute excellent and expedient review sources. If you did not make summaries, then you should select review books that include lots of charts, diagrams, or any other forms of review that highlight important relationships among concepts (see Chapter 3).

4. **Cramming interferes with memory processes.** Attempting to learn large amounts of material in a very short time leads to confusion and forgetting. Even though cramming may have resulted in reasonable (possibly good) grades on examinations during medical school courses, it is a study method that does not yield very good long-term retention. Topics that you learned by cramming will require much more effort and time to review than subjects that were studied at a regular, steady pace. Be sure to start your USMLE review early to minimize addi-

tional confusion and forgetting (see Chapter 7) and spend more time reviewing those courses in which you used cramming.

5. **Spaced learning improves memory savings.** In other words, everything reviewed today will take less time to refresh in memory just before examinations. Leaving things until the last minute is **not** an effective means of preventing forgetting. As we discussed above, the act of cramming itself causes memory interference. If material is reviewed effectively, then even when it seems forgotten, it can be refreshed rapidly and with minimum effort just before exams. So don't wait until the last minute to begin reviewing; start as early as you can, since every little bit of review will pay off in the end.

6. **Intermittent review helps protect against forgetting** and promotes the transfer of knowledge to long-term memory. The only way to guard against forgetting is to intermittently review the material and to identify and relearn topics that have been subject to the greatest forgetting.

7. **Frequent self-testing identifies topics most prone to forgetting.** Self-testing also helps maintain knowledge by acting to refresh your memory. Even well-learned material can be subject to forgetting. Therefore, to determine if and what knowledge you might be forgetting, quiz yourself regularly. As you review for USMLE, you will find using the practice examinations presented in Chapter 5 very helpful.

Familiarity should not be equated with knowing
Understanding increases memory retention
Active learning greatly increases subsequent recall
Cramming interferes with memory processes
Spaced learning improves memory savings
Intermittent review helps protect against forgetting
Frequent self-testing identifies topics prone to forgetting

Identify Your Most Forgetting-Prone Topics

Consider each basic science and make a list of topics that:

- you didn't understand well initially
- you learned by cramming
- you learned by rote or passively
- you have not reviewed recently in current courses

Anatomy

Behavioral Science

Biochemistry

Pathology

Pharmacology

Physiology

Microbiology

The topics you have just listed will probably require more time and effort to review than others. Consider this list when constructing your USMLE Review Plan in Chapter 7. Begin your review with your most difficult subjects.

Chapter 3

What Resources to Use and When and How to Use Them

This chapter discusses how to select among the myriad review materials available for USMLE preparation, and how to use these resources efficiently and effectively.

SELECTING REVIEW MATERIALS There are a great number of review materials presenting essential summaries of the basic science material that is addressed on the USMLE. Selecting among these frequently presents a major challenge since the format, length, amount of detail, and organization can vary greatly from one to the next. In addition, students who have already taken the examination may provide an abundance of conflicting recommendations about which sources are best that can further complicate the selection process.

INFORMATION SOURCES

—one (and only one) condensed summary of each subject (e.g., class notes, commercial review books)

—one or more board-type practice question books for each subject, organized by subtopics, with complete explanations

—one major textbook for each science, to be used only as a back-up if parts of the review book don't meet your needs

---

In choosing review materials, it is extremely important to remember that what might have been an excellent source for one individual can be inappropriate for another. So don't blindly accept the advice of your peers; instead, critically evaluate the sources available to you and choose materials to suit your individual needs and learning style. The following guidelines should help you decide what materials you will be able to use most efficiently and effectively. Effective USMLE preparation requires three types of sources: a **summary**, **practice questions**, and a **major textbook**.

SELECTING A SUMMARY SOURCE In evaluating and selecting a summary source for review of each science consider the following:

FORMAT Is the format of the source consistent with your preference? Some review materials are presented primarily in <u>outline</u> <u>format</u> (e.g., Stanley Kaplan Review Books), while others are written in <u>prose</u> (e.g., A. Little Brown Book Series, Rypin's Guide to Medical Licensure). Yet others are more of a mixture of these two forms (e.g., National Medical Series Review Books Board Review Series, Oklahoma Notes Series). Choose a format that suits your learning style. Different sciences may require different formats: for example, you may find it easier to review physiology when it is presented in full sentences as opposed to outline format, while the opposite may be true of pharmacology.

FAMILIARITY Have you used the source before? A familiar source is faster and easier to use than an unfamiliar source. If you used (and liked) a particular commercial review book to accompany your studies in medical school, stick with it for USMLE review. However, it is not necessary to use commercial review books for all, or any, basic sciences: if you have a set of class notes or faculty prepared notes that you used as primary study source in medical school, by all means use this for your USMLE review.

CHARTS, DIAGRAMS, ETC. Does the source you have chosen include lots of good charts, diagrams, and/or pictures that highlight important relationships? Charts, diagrams, flowcharts, and drawings comprise some of the best ways to summarize complex and detailed topics. Any source that makes extensive use of these devices can make reviewing much more efficient, (e.g., Pharmacology: *MedCharts)*. If you made charts and other essential summaries during medical school, be sure to use these to supplement your USMLE review.

DETAIL Is the source sufficiently detailed for your needs? Consider your competence in an area when you are selecting a review book. If you feel relatively weak in a particular subject, beware of choosing a review source that is too list-like, since you may have difficulty understanding the material. Instead, be sure that the review has enough explanatory text so you can make sense of it. A more cryptic review may be adequate for your stronger subjects.

LENGTH Is it an appropriate length, given the number of days that you can realistically devote to studying the subject? Review materials can vary enormously in length. While it is important not to choose one that is so brief that you cannot understand it, you should also avoid materials that are too detailed and extensive to be covered in the time you have available for study. Be sure to consider the type-size, the margin space, and the amount of actual text (as opposed to charts and diagrams), and not just the number of pages, in determining the actual length of the review. An excellent source may be overlooked because at a glance it appears to be too lengthy.

SELECTING A USMLE PRACTICE QUESTION SOURCE A practice question book is an invaluable and critical component of effective USMLE preparation. Practice questions serve many important functions (see Chapter 4) and they should be used in a regular, intermittent fashion as part of every study plan.

HOW TO EVALUATE QUESTION SOURCES

—Is it organized by subtopics within each basic science? Question books which are not organized this way cannot be used to enhance the study process.

—Is it designed to reflect the content emphasis, difficulty level, and question types of the USMLE?

—Does it have comprehensive explanations for each question? A comprehensive explanation should be referenced and provide information about both the correct and the incorrect answers. Books which do not explain **why** the wrong answers are wrong are of limited value.

—The PreTest® books in this series are designed to meet all of these requirements.

SELECTING A MAJOR TEXT Since it is not possible to know whether the review book you have selected will meet your needs completely, it is important to have a good comprehensive textbook on hand to fill in gaps when (and if) needed. The textbooks that you used during medical school will likely suit your needs. The references supplied in the practice question books provide good alternates.

REVIEW METHOD Many students assume that a quick, superficial reading of the review materials from beginning to end is an adequate "memory refresher" for USMLE preparation. Others decide that a selective review of just a few weak topics within each science is satisfactory. Still others choose to focus on their areas of greatest strength, reasoning that they will be able to compensate for weaknesses by being especially proficient in certain areas. Although these approaches may require little time, none of them is likely to be particularly productive. An approach that will yield the greatest gains should be both comprehensive and tailored to your own particular strengths and weaknesses.

Comprehensive Neglecting certain topics can result in very disappointing USMLE scores. This is because even if you were to answer every question correctly on a selection of topics (even half of the topics covered on the exam), you would probably only achieve a score of 50% which is not sufficient to pass. Even with the most impressive review approach, your chances of correctly answering every question on a selection of topics is very remote.

Tailored Your weakest topics should receive more time and effort than your stronger subjects. However, your strongest subjects should not be neglected entirely; a cursory, but active, review should suffice in these areas. There is a law of diminishing returns when it comes to reviewing for the USMLE: the better you know the material, the less you stand to gain by investing a lot of time reviewing. Conversely, the less well you know the material, the more you can gain by study.

SOME GOOD ADVICE

—Passive reading of your review materials may trigger memories momentarily but will not yield good long-term recall and will not promote good problem-solving skills.

—Be certain that you test your ability to recall, as opposed to recognize, material as you review.

—Make use of practice questions on a regular basis to ensure that you can recall and apply the material.

GENERAL GUIDELINES FOR APPROACHING REVIEW MATERIALS

Step 1. Quickly overview the headings within a chapter or set of notes so you will know what to expect in the section.

Step 2. Read any introductory remarks so you will be mentally oriented for what is to come.

Step 3. Skim a subsection to get a sense of what details are covered in the section.

Step 4. Cover the section with your hands, and try to recall as much as you can. Write down key words or make brief notes.

Step 5. Skim the section again, slowing down to read and think about information that you didn't remember, don't know, or remember incorrectly; highlight these items. Don't bother highlighting material that you accurately recall.

Step 6. Work through every section in the chapter or your notes by repeating steps 3 through 5 for each one.

Step 7. When you have completed an entire chapter, test your ability to recall and apply the information by using USMLE review questions (see Chapter 4 for specific suggestions).

Step 8. Upgrade your knowledge and focus additional review as indicated by your performance on questions.

Chapter 4

Why Use Questions and How to Use Them

This chapter explains how to properly use books of questions and practice examinations.

OVERVIEW Students preparing for the licensing examinations frequently underestimate the enormous value of practice questions. Practice questions serve many important functions and may be used in many different ways throughout the review process. This chapter discusses how to use questions most effectively. Notice that they have uses before, during, and after review.

USING QUESTIONS BEFORE REVIEW Even before you begin to review, practice questions can be used to help answer three important questions.

1. How should your review be focused?

Read through practice questions in a section of a review book, without trying to answer them. This will help you to develop a sense of the content, difficulty, and level of integration that is required on the USMLE, and thus help you determine an effective approach to study.

For example, by reading questions in the Anatomy PreTest®, you learn that you must know the brachial plexus in detail (all its branches and subbranches), not just in general terms. In addition, you find that you must be able to apply your knowledge to clinical situations, to group nerves by their functions, and to compare and contrast the functions of various muscles groups. Other insights of this type can be gleaned by reading questions ahead of your review so you can ensure that your study approach is appropriate to the demands of the questions.

2. How much review is needed in each topic?

Testing yourself before any review can determine how much additional study is necessary in each science to achieve your goal. Remember that you must correctly answer about 55-60 percent of the questions to pass the exam. Scores below 50 percent indicate that organized, comprehensive study is required. For your convenience, in chapter 5 we have constructed comprehensive self-tests of 25 questions in each basic science that you could use for this purpose. These tests are based on a careful, balanced selection of questions from each of the PreTest® Self-Assessment and Review books. Further instructions on how to use these tests are provided later in this chapter, and answers and subtopic classifications are found in the Appendix.

3. What are your strengths and weaknesses?

After taking a self-test and before studying, look at your pattern of errors to determine what specific subtopics require the most study. For example, you may discover that a disproportionate number of your errors in pharmacology were related to cardiovascular and endocrine drugs, but that you did fairly well on questions about other classes of drugs. Alternatively, you may discover that your errors were evenly divided across classes of drugs, but that you made more errors when the questions were related to drug mechanisms than when related to drug uses and side effects. This pattern suggests that you need to pay particular attention to drug mechanisms as you study. In either case, it is clear that you can invest your limited time most productively if you are aware of where the greatest payoffs will be.

Before you start studying:

–read questions to develop an appropriate focus for your review

–take a pre-test (25 questions) to determine how much review is required to achieve your goals

–look at your pattern of errors to determine your strengths and weaknesses

---

USING QUESTIONS DURING REVIEW Continue to use practice questions as an integral part of your review program. Doing questions can help transfer information to long-term memory. Test yourself each time you finish reviewing a major subtopic within each science. The PreTest® question books are organized by subtopics for easy use in this manner. Practice questions used regularly as you review can help answer all the following questions:

---

1. Do you know enough to pass the exam?

Take practice exams to determine whether or not you have mastered the material at a sufficient level of detail and understanding to pass the actual examination. Our experience with the PreTest® questions leads us to believe that scores averaging 60 percent or better on these practice exams indicate a sufficient mastery of the material to pass the USMLE. Don't forget, however, about forgetting (see Chapter 2).

---

2. Is your review source adequate?

If you get a number of questions wrong because the material is not covered in your review book (be sure to check), you may need to use another review source for selected topics.

---

3. Is your study style effective?

If you get questions wrong, and the material is actually covered in your review source (be sure to check), you need to revise your study approach. Don't blindly assume that your errors mean that your review book is unsatisfactory. It could be your approach.

---

4. What topics require additional review?

You may discover that most of your errors cluster around certain topics. If so, you need more review time in those areas.

> 5. Can you use your knowledge to solve problems?

Just because you have reviewed and memorized does not guarantee that you can apply your knowledge to solve problems. This is a particularly important reason to use practice questions, since the board examination emphasizes problem solving and integration of knowledge. Study as if for an essay exam.

> 6. Do you have effective test-taking skills?

You may discover that many of your mistakes are due to carelessness, or that your pacing is not up to par. If so, continue to use questions to help you develop good test-taking strategies (see Chapter 8).

USING QUESTIONS AFTER REVIEW Once you have completed your primary review of a basic science, take a comprehensive post-test to determine your level of proficiency. The comprehensive practice tests in the next chapter can be used for this purpose. Continue to use questions intermittently to help detect and guard against forgetting. The explanations provided in the PreTest® books can be used to refresh and upgrade your knowledge in deficient areas. Be sure that you understand why the incorrect alternatives are wrong when you review your answers.

On the next page is a method that should help you get the most out of practice questions after your review of a subject.

Using Practice Questions

1. Take a practice test when you feel that you have adequately reviewed the material for a specific topic. Twenty to thirty questions should suffice for a subtopic. Do every second or third question if there are a large number of questions for a section. Save the others for additional self-testing and review at a later time.

2. Time yourself, allowing 55 seconds per question.

3. Each time you select an answer to a question, indicate how confident you are about your answer using the following codes:

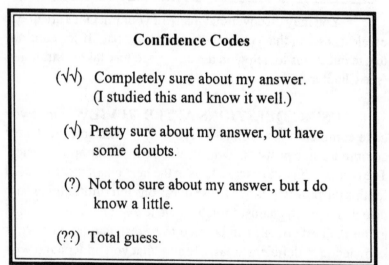

Confidence Codes

(√√)   Completely sure about my answer. (I studied this and know it well.)

(√)   Pretty sure about my answer, but have some doubts.

(?)   Not too sure about my answer, but I do know a little.

(??)   Total guess.

Don't omit this step. It takes little extra time and it will help you determine how often you make careless errors (usually when you are pretty confident). It will also prevent you from failing to learn from questions that you may get right through guess work (correct answers selected but with low confidence).

4. When you have completed the test, grade it, but don't look up the correct answers yet. Pay close attention to the relationship between your errors and your confidence ratings as described below.

5. Now return to any questions you got wrong in the completely sure confidence category ($\sqrt{\sqrt{}}$). Reread each question, rethink, and try to figure out what the correct answer should be. Maybe you made a careless error if you were highly confident. How can you avoid this error in the future: Did you fail to read all of the alternatives? Did you misinterpret the questions? etc. Even a few errors (1 or 2) when you are highly confident can seriously compromise your performance on the USMLE.

6. Follow the procedure outlined previously (5) for errors you made when you were Pretty Sure ($\sqrt{}$). Errors in this confidence category may reflect poor deductive reasoning skills (see the section in Chapter 7 on deductive reasoning under uncertainty).

7. Review questions and explanations for errors that you made in both low confidence categories (? and ??) to upgrade your knowledge. There is not much point retrying these questions since you probably just don't know enough. Return to your review book if necessary for certain topics. If you have used these low confidence ratings for more than 15-20% of the questions in a given test, it is likely that your study approach requires modification. A large number of "total guesses" (??) may mean your review is deficient. A large number of "Not too sures" (?) may mean your review method is too passive. (see Chapter 3)

8. Review questions and explanations for those you answered correctly in the low confidence categories. Since, with these questions, you may have been correct solely on the basis of

chance, don't give yourself credit for these lucky accidents when preparing for the licensing examination. Instead, go back and try to learn more about the related topics.

9. Check your errors and low confidence questions to see if there is a pattern indicating some specific topic or topics that could benefit from additional study.

HOW TO EVALUATE REVIEW SOURCES

—Select a <u>small</u> topic that you need to review.

—Study or survey the relevant section in the review source.

—Try to answer questions related to the topic in a practice question book (e.g., PreTest®). (If you are sampling a commercially prepared review book, it is best to use questions prepared by a different publisher. This is because the questions included in the review books themselves may use the same wording as the text, making them easier to answer, and possibly leading to the false impression that the review book meets your needs.)

—If information necessary to answer the questions is presented clearly in the review source, it is likely to be adequate for you.

PRACTICE EXAMINATIONS In the following chapter, we have constructed two comprehensive tests in each basic science based on a careful selection of questions from the PreTest® review books. You may want to use one as a pre-test and the other as a post-test as described earlier. We have also included one practice exam in Genetics and another in Neuroscience since these subjects are often taught as separate courses and you may be reviewing them as discrete units. We have indicated the topic of each question in the Appendix. Find the correct answers in the Appendix as well.

Chapter 5

Practice Tests

This chapter contains 16 25-question practice tests.

OVERVIEW Use these practice tests before and after you have reviewed each subject as described in Chapter 4.

PRACTICE TESTS To use the following exams, carefully cut out the answer sheet and enter your answers (ANS) and confidence rating (CON) in the spaces provided. We suggest that you use the first exam **before** you begin your review of the subject. It will provide you with some idea of how much review will be required and in which specific subtopics. Use the second practice exam after you have reviewed to determine how effective your review has been and what additional studying you may need to do.

Remember to time yourself when you are taking these exams. These practice exams should require no more than 25 minutes each. Doing them in twenty minutes would be better.

When you have completed the exam, turn to the Appendix and mark each question you answered incorrectly. Count the number of question you answered correctly and divide that number by 25 (the total number of questions on the exam). Multiply by 100 and the result is your score (percent correct). You should get at least 65 percent correct.

Finally, note the subtopics of the questions you missed and be sure to undertake additional review in those areas.

TABLE OF CONTENTS FOR THE PRACTICE TESTS

COMMENTS ABOUT THE PRACTICE TESTS

When evaluating your performance on these practice examinations, you should keep the following in mind:

1. Scores of 65 percent or better suggest sufficient knowledge to pass the USMLE.
2. Scores of 60 to 65 percent are marginal.
3. Scores of less than 55 percent indicate that further study is required.

ANATOMY I PRACTICE TEST

ANSWER SHEET

	ANS	CON
1.		
2.		
3.		
4.		
5.		
6.		
7.		
8.		
9.		
10.		
11.		
12.		
13.		

	ANS	CON
14.		
15.		
16.		
17.		
18.		
19.		
20.		
21.		
22.		
23.		
24.		
25.		

CUT HERE

SEE PAGE 25 FOR INSTRUCTIONS
SEE PAGE 211 FOR ANSWERS

STUDY SUGGESTION

As you review facts and concepts, consider them in terms of organizational levels. Remember, the USMLE will present questions apportioned to the major levels of organization as below:

15-25% – Person (e.g., society, family, individual)

50-60% – Organ/tissue,
Cell/subcellular,
Molecular

15-25% – Nonhuman organism,
Exogenous substance

ANATOMY I

1. By the process of induction, certain embryonic tissues alter the microenvironment of adjacent cells and tissues. Examples of induction during embryogenesis include development of all the following structures EXCEPT the

(A) adenohypophysis by neural ectoderm

(B) lens by the optic vesicle

(C) mammary gland by the underlying mesoderm

(D) mesenchyme of a limb by the apical ectodermal ridge

(E) neural plate by brain and notochord

2. A common developmental pattern shared by sebaceous glands, sweat glands, mammary glands, hair follicles, and nails is

(A) development from neural crest cells

(B) derivation from mesenchyme

(C) differentiation influenced by steroids

(D) invagination of epidermal cells into the dermis

(E) none of the above

3. A factor applicable to both skeletal and smooth muscles is

(A) a system of T-tubules that conveys the membrane depolarization deep into the cell

(B) contraction regulated by controlling intracellular calcium concentration

(C) gap junctions that spread membrane depolarizations to adjacent fibers

(D) innervation that is generally by motor neurons that lie in the anterior horn of the spinal cord

(E) intercalated disks that serve as anchoring locations for thin filaments

4. A symptom complex of dysphagia, dysphonia with deviation of the palate to the left, and hoarseness caused by adduction of the right vocal cords is due to involvement of which nerve(s)?

(A) Left glossopharyngeal nerve

(B) Left vagus nerve

(C) Left vagus AND left glossopharyngeal

(D) Right glossopharyngeal nerve

(E) Right vagus nerve

5. During anesthesia-induced muscle relaxation, obstruction of the respiratory passage is prevented by forward traction on the mandible. Normally, the tongue is prevented from falling backward and obstructing respiration by the

(A) genioglossus muscle

(B) hyoglossus muscle

(C) mylohyoid muscle

(D) palatoglossus muscle

(E) styloglossus muscle

6. The cells of the nephron have distinctive structures that subserve different functions. Correct statements include all the following EXCEPT

(A) the cells of the proximal convoluted tubule have a brush border (numerous microvilli) that provides an increased absorptive surface

(B) the cells of the visceral layer of Bowman's capsule (podocytes) act variably as a barrier to filtration

(C) the cuboidal cells of the collecting tubules are responsive to hormones that determine their permeability to water

(D) the macula densa is a modification of the distal convoluted tubule

(E) the squamous cells of the descending limb of the loop of Henle are impermeable to water

7. A cell that is extensively involved in protein synthesis and exocytosis is:

(A) Monocyte

(B) Platelet

(C) Eosinophil

(D) Neutrophil

(E) Plasma cell

8. A 23 -year-old, semiconscious man is brought to the emergency room following an automobile accident. He is tachypneic (breathing rapidly) and cyanotic (blue lips and nail beds). The right lower anterolateral thoracic wall reveals a small laceration and flailing (moving *inward* as the rest of the thoracic cage expands during inspira-tion). Air does not appear to move into or out of the wound, and it is assumed that the pleura has not been penetrated. After the patient is placed on immediate positive pressure endotracheal respiration, his cyanosis clears and the abnormal movement of the chest wall diappears. Radiographic examination confirms fractures of the fourth through eighth ribs in the right anteroaxillary line and of the fourth through sixth ribs at the right costochondral junction. There is no evidence that bony fragments have penetrated the lungs or of pneumothorax (collapsed lung). In this patient, the initial cyanosis - incomplete oxygenation of the blood owing to perfusion of the right lung without ventilation - is a result of

(A) bilateral inability of the pleural cavaties to expand

(B) inability of the right chest wall to expand the pleural cavity

(C) paralysis of the right hemidiaphragm

(D) paralysis of the thoracic musculature

(E) shunting of all blood through the normal lung

9. Knowledge of the lymphatic drainage of the breast is clinically important because of the high incidence of breast tumors. The major pathway of lymphatic drainage from the mammary gland is along lymphatic channels that parallel

(A) subcutaneous venous networks to the contralateral breast and to the abdominal wall

(B) tributaries of the axillary vessels to the axillary nodes

(C) tributaries of the intercostal vessels to the parasternal nodes and posterior mediastinal nodes

(D) tributaries of the internal thoracic (mammary) vessels to the paraster-nal (internal thoracic) nodes

(E) tributaries of the thoracoacromial vessels to the apical (subclavicular) nodes

10. A posteriorly perforating ulcer in the pyloric antrum of the stomach is most likely to produce initial localized peritonitis or abscess formation in the

(A) greater sac

(B) left subhepatic and hepatorenal spaces (pouch of Morison)

(C) omental bursa

(D) right subphrenic space

(E) right subhepatic space

11. In addition to the vas deferens, structures normally found within the internal spermatic fascia of the spermatic cord include all the following EXCEPT the

(A) deferential artery

(B) ilioinguinal nerve

(C) pampiniform plexus

(D) testicular artery

(E) testicular nerve

12. In angina pectoris, the pain radiating down the left arm is mediated by increased activity in afferent (sensory) fibers contained in

(A) the carotid branch of the glossopharyngeal nerves

(B) the greater splanchinic nerves

(C) the phrenic nerves

(D) the vagus and recurrent laryngeal nerves

(E) the sympathetic cervical and thoracic cardiac fibers

13. Pain associated with external hemorrhoids is mediated by

(A) the hypogastric nerves to the lumbar splanchnic nerves

(B) the pelvic splanchnic nerves (nervi erigentes)

(C) the pudenal nerve

(D) the sacral sympathetic chain

(E) none of the above

14. An inguinal, rather than a femoral, hernia is suspected in this patient for all the following reasons EXCEPT

(A) the bulge begins superior to the inguinal ligament

(B) the bulge occurs midway between the symphysis pubis and anterior superior iliac spine

(C) femoral hernias occur only in females

(D) the hernia extends into the superior portion of the scrotal sac

15. Fibers of the optic tract terminate in

(A) the inferior corpus quadrigeminus (colliculus)

(B) the lateral geniculate body

(C) the medial geniculate body

(D) the ventral posteromedial nucleus of the thalamus

(E) none of the above

16. The principle efferent pathway from the hippocampus is the

(A) alvear pathway

(B) fornix

(C) medial forebrain bundle

(D) perforant pathway

(E) stria terminalis

17. A 24-year-old woman seeking assistance for apparent infertility has been unable to conceive in spite of repeated attempts in 5 years of marriage. She revealed that her husband had fathered a child in a prior marriage. Although the patient's menstrual periods are fairly regular, they are accompanied by extreme low back pain. The low back pain during menstruation experienced by the woman described probably is referred from the pelvic region. The pathways that convey this pain sensation to the central nervous system involve

(A) the hypogastric nerve to L1-L2.

(B) the lumbosacral trunk to L4-L5

(C) the nervi erigentes (pelvic nerve) to S2-S4

(D) the pudendal nerve to S2-S4

(E) none of the above

18. The following pelvic structures are correctly linked to the somatic regions to which they refer pain EXCEPT

(A) the cervix to the perineum, leg, and foot

(B) the epididymis to the lumbar and umbilical regions

(C) the mid-ureter to the inguinal region, pubic region, and medial thigh

(D) the ovary to the umbilical region, lumbar region, and medial thigh

(E) the uterine body to the inguinal region, hypogastric region, and medial thigh

19. A man who has a deep laceration of the scalp with profuse bleeding is seen in the emergency room. His epicranial aponeurosis(galeo aponeurotica) is penetrated, resulting in severe gaping of the wound. The structure underlying the epicranial aponeurosis is
(A) a layer containing blood vessels
(B) bone
(C) the dura mater
(D) the periosteum (pericranium)
(E) the tendon of the epicranial muscles (occipitofrontalis)

20. The observation that extension at the elbow appears normal, but supination of the forearm weak, warrants localization of the nerve lesion to the
(A) posterior cord of the brachial plexus in the axilla
(B) posterior division of brachial plexus
(C) radial nerve at distal third of humerus
(D) radial nerve in the midforearm
(E) radial nerve in vicinity of the head of the radius

21. As a result of automotive trauma, a person sustains a complete crush-injury of the right half of the spinal cord(Brown-Sequard's syndrome) at the T12 level. Findings at neurologic examination include
(A) contralateral flaccid paralysis at the level of the lesion
(B) contralateral loss of position sense and two-point discrimination below lesion
(C) contralateral loss of light touch below the lesion
(D) ipsilateral loss of pain and temperature below the lesion
(E) ipsilateral motor paralysis with spasticity below the lesion

22. Like all endocrine glands, the thyroid is highly vascular. The thyroid gland receives its blood supply in part from the branches of the
(A) internal carotid artery
(B) lingual artery
(C) subclavian artery
(D) transverse cervical artery

23. Lumbar vertebrae are characterized by all the following EXCEPT
(A) a large and heavy body
(B) articular surfaces that permit little rotation
(C) deep intervertebral notches in the inferior surfaces of the pedicles
(D) greater thickness anteriorly than posteriorly to provide the lumbar curvature
(E) short, broad, horizontal spinous processes

24. Protein translocation across the membrane of endoplasmic reticulum involves a signal peptide, a signal-recognition particle, and a signal-recognition particle receptor. All the following statements are correct regarding the signal peptide EXCEPT
(A) it bonds directly to the signal-recognition particle receptor
(B) it is associated only with peptides destined for export
(C) it is cleaved from the peptide before the peptide is fully synthesized
(D) it is found within the endoplasmic reticulum
(E) it is located at the N-terminal of the synthesized peptide

25. Reflexes that protect the inner ear from excessive noise involve the contraction of the tensor tympani and stapedius muscles. Correct statements about the tensor tympani muscle include all the following EXCEPT

(A) it inserts onto the malleus

(B) it is derived from the first branchial arch

(C) it is innervated by the chorda tympani nerve

(D) it lies parallel to the auditory tube

STUDY SUGGESTION

Does your Review Plan need to be modified? Are you behind (or ahead of) schedule? If you have not accomplished everything you had planned up until this point, take 30 minutes to reconstruct your plan.

ANATOMY II PRACTICE TEST

ANSWER SHEET

CUT HERE

	ANS	CON		ANS	CON
1.			14.		
2.			15.		
3.			16.		
4.			17.		
5.			18.		
6.			19.		
7.			20.		
8.			21.		
9.			22.		
10.			23.		
11.			24.		
12.			25.		
13.					

SEE PAGE 25 FOR INSTRUCTIONS
SEE PAGE 211 FOR ANSWERS

STUDY SUGGESTION

Have you taken several practice question tests by now? If not, how can you be sure your review program has the appropriate emphasis, and that your review is productive? (Return to Chapter 4.)

ANATOMY II

1. All the following statements concerning the acrosome reaction are correct EXCEPT

(A) it injects the contents of the acrosomal envelope into the cytoplasm of the egg

(B) it involves the formation of the acrosomal process

(C) it releases acid hydrolases onto the zona pellucida

(D) it terminates upon fusion of the plasma membrane of the sperm with that of the egg

(E) it triggers fusion of the outer acrosomal membrane with the plasma membrane of the sperm

2. The skeletal and connective tissue structures of the lower portion of the face and anterior neck are derived from neural crest cells in the branchial arches. All the following structures derive from the second branchial arch EXCEPT the

(A) lesser horn of the hyoid bone

(B) malleus

(C) stapes

(D) styloid process of the temporal bone

(E) stylohyoid ligament

3. Regions of the retina that contain rod cells include

(A) the fovea centralis

(B) the macula lutea

(C) the optic disk

(D) the ora serrata

(E) none of the above

4. The culture is incubated (pulsed) in a medium containing ^{3}H-thymidine for exactly 2 hours. Subsequently, the culture is incubated (chased) in a medium containing nonradioactive thymidine for exactly 1 hour. The cells are then fixed and prepared for radioautography. On exam-ination with a light microscope, silver grains exposed by incorporated radioactivity are observed over a small percentage of nuclei. Which of the following conclusions is correct?

(A) Labeled cells are daughter cells with a 2n chromosome number

(B) Labeled cells were fixed when they were in the S phase of the cell cycle

(C) Labeled cells were in the S phase of the cell cycle during the pulse of ^{3}H-thymidine

(D) Unlabeled cells are incapable of gene replication and are not part of the cycling population of cells

(E) None of the above

5. Filaments of actin and myosin compose the contractile apparatus in striated muscle. All the following statements about the myofilaments are correct EXCEPT

(A) the A-band lattice is a liquid-crystalline structure

(B) the actin filament is a triple helix of globular actin monomers

(C) the myosin heads undergo conformational changes when they bind to actin

(D) the parallel array of myosin filaments is strongly anisotropic in polarized light

(E) the thick filaments are composed of molecules having a structure similar to an antibody

6. In gametogenesis, meiosis differs significantly from mitosis. All the following are characteristics of meiosis EXCEPT

(A) crossing-over occurs between sister chromatids during prophase I

(B) daughter cells enter a second M phase of the cell cycle after division I without passing through the G_1 phase and S phase

(C) independent assortment of maternal and paternal genetic material occurs in division I

(D) the result of division I is a chromosomal reduction to the haploid number

(E) there is pairing of homologous chromosomes

7. Select the principle collagen found in loose connective tissue and blood vessels.

(A) Type I collagen

(B) Type II collagen

(C) Type III collagen

(D) Type IV collagen

(E) Type V collagen

8. One liter of blood is withdrawn from the pleural cavity; the patient's cyanosis immediately clears and signs of the mediastinal shift disappear. Possible sources of the bleeding that produces the hemothorax include all the following EXCEPT the

(A) intercostal arteries

(B) internal thoracic artery

(C) lateral thoracic artery

(D) musculophrenic artery

(E) vessels associated with the lung parenchyma

9. A middle-aged woman describes flushing, severe headaches, and a feeling that her heart is "going to explode" when she gets excited. At the beginning of a physical examination her blood pressure (130/85) is not significantly above normal. However, upon palpation of her upper left quadrant the examining physician notices the onset of sympathetic signs. Her blood pressure (200/135) is abnormally high. A subsequent CT scan confirms the suspected tumor of the left adrenal gland. The patient is scheduled for surgery. The symptoms that the patient correlated with the onset of excitement were due to nervous stimulation of the adrenal glands. The adrenal medulla receives its innervation from

(A) preganglionic sympathetic nerves

(B) postsynaptic sympathetic nerves

(C) preganglionic parasympathetic nerves

(D) postganglionic parasympathetic nerves

(E) somatic nerves

10. All the following statements correctly characterize the pelvic diaphragm, which forms the floor of the abdominopelvic cavity, EXCEPT

(A) it comprises the levator ani and coccygeus muscles with their fascia

(B) it functions to support the pelvic organs

(C) it is innervated by twigs from the sacral plexus

(D) it lies in the same plane as the urogenital diaphragm

(E) it originates in part from a condensation of fascia across the obturator internis muscle

11. The blood supply to the ureters is derived from all the following arteries EXCEPT the

(A) common iliac

(B) gonadal

(C) inferior mesenteric

(D) inferior vesical

(E) renal

12. Select the appropriate male homologue for the female pelvic structure, the vestibule

(A) Corpus spongiosum

(B) Scrotum

(C) Scrotal raphe

(D) Penile (cavernous) urethra

(E) None of the above

13. A 53-year-old woman has a paralysis of the right side of her face that produces an expressionless and drooping appearance. She is unable to close her right eye, has difficulty chewing and drinking, perceives sounds as annoyingly intense in her right ear, and experiences some pain in her right external auditory meatus. Physical examination reveals loss of blink reflex in the right eye upon stimulation of either cornea and loss of taste from the anterior two-thirds of the tongue on the right side. Lacrimation appears normal in the right eye, the jawjerk reflex is normal, and there appears to be no problem with balance. The inability to close the right eye is the result of involvement of

(A) the buccal branch of the facial nerve

(B) the buccal branch of the trigeminal nerve

(C) the levator palpebrae superioris muscle

(D) the superior tarsal muscle (of Müller)

(E) none of the above

14. Infection of the angular vein may result in venous thrombosis in which of the following intracranial vessels?

(A) Cavernous sinus

(B) Inferior petrosal sinus

(C) Sagittal sinus

(D) Sigmoid sinus

(E) Sphenoid sinus

15. A child suspected of aspirating a small cloth-covered metal button is seen in the emergency room. While the child does not complain of pain, there is frequent coughing. Anticipating absence of breath sounds, the examining physician listens with a stethoscope to the right lung. Aspirated small objects tend to lodge in the right inferior lobar bronchus for all the following reasons EXCEPT

(A) the left main stem (primary) bronchus is more horizontal than the right

(B) the right inferior lobar bronchus nearly continues the direction of the trachea

(C) the right lung has no middle lobe

(D) the right main stem (primary) bronchus is of greater diameter than the left

16. Injury to the posterior cord of the brachial plexus involves all the following nerves EXCEPT the

(A) axillary nerve

(B) long thoracic nerve

(C) radial nerve

(D) subscapular nerves

(E) thoracodorsal nerve

17. When the interior of the mouth is examined and the patient asked to say AH-H-H-H, the palate is observed to deviate to the normal side and there is loss of the gag reflex on the injured side. From these observations, it can be determined that all the following muscles are paralyzed on the injured side EXCEPT the

(A) levator veli palatini

(B) palatopharyngeus

(C) stylohyoid

(D) stylopharyngeus

(E) superior pharyngeal constrictor

18. The patterns for both containment and spread of infection within the palmar anatomic spaces of the hand are explained by all the following relationships EXCEPT

(A) the synovial sheath of the flexor pollicis longus (radial bursa) extends through the palm to the distal phalanx of the thumb the

(B) common tendon sheath (bursa), containing the flexor tendons of the second, third, and fourth digits, extends through the palm to the distal phalanges

(C) the synovial sheath of the flexor tendons of the fifth digit (ulnar bursa) extends through the palm to the distal phalanx

(D) the radial, ulnar, and common bursas extend beneath the flexor retinaculum into the wrist

(E) the radial and ulnar bursas may communicate with the common tendon sheath

19. Articulation of the talus with the malleoli and lower tibia forms the ankle, or talocrural, joint. Factors that contribute to the stability of this joint include all the following EXCEPT the

(A) calcaneonavicular ("spring") ligament

(B) deltoid ligament

(C) lateral ligament

(D) posterior tibiofibular ligament

(E) trapezoidal shape of the talar articular surface (wider anteriorly than posteriorly)

20. A woman comes to the emergency room after sustaining a severe burn on her left hand. She was unaware of the injury until the burn area was observed. Neurologic examination reveals a bilateral dissociated sensory loss (absence or impairment of pain and temperature sense with nearly normal tactile pressure and position sense) over most of the left and right upper extremities and first thoracic dermatome of the chest. Above and below a shawl-like region about the shoulders, all sensory modalities are normal

In the patient presented, the lesion most probably involves the

(A) anterior white commissure

(B) dorsal horn

(C) dorsal nucleus (of Clarke)

(D) dorsolateral funiculus

(E) posterior funiculus

21. In this patient, paralysis of the left facial nerve accounts for all the following EXCEPT

(A) hyperacusis on the left side

(B) loss of the corneal blink reflex

(C) loss of left lacrimal gland secretion

(D) loss of left parotid gland secretion

(E) loss of taste from the left anterior two-thirds of the tongue

22. A stroke involving the amygdaloid body of the limbic system results in aberrations in all the following EXCEPT

(A) hypophyseal hormone secretion

(B) intelligence

(C) sex drive

(D) temperament

(E) visceral autonomic responses

23. Cerebrospinal fluid directly enters the cisterna magna

(A) at arachnoid granulations

(B) from the choroid plexus

(C) through the foramina of Luschka and Magendie

(D) through the foramina of Monro

(E) via the iter of Sylvius (cerebral aqueduct)

24. Sympathetic and parasympathetic nerves reach the pelvic plexus by different pathways. During surgical resection of the rectum, the sympathetic nerves had to be excised bilaterally, leading to which of the following complications?

(A) A dilated and neurogenic bladder

(B) Loss of control of the external urethral sphincter

(C) Impotence (inability to obtain erection)

(D) Inability to ejaculate

(E) None of the above

25. In the extended position, the knee becomes rigid and stable because the medial femoral condyle rides posteriorly and on the tibial plateau, rotating the femur medially or the tibia laterally and achieving a configuration that effectively "locks" the knee. The process of "unlocking" the knee in preparation for flexion requires initial contraction of the

(A) gastrocnemius, soleus, and plantaris muscles

(B) hamstring muscles

(C) popliteus muscle

(D) quadriceps femoris muscle

(E) sartorius muscle and short head of the biceps femoris muscle

STUDY SUGGESTION

Don't anguish over selecting the perfect source for review. Chapter 3 can help you choose ones that suit your needs. Stick with whatever you've selected. Every source has strengths and weaknesses. Practice questions will help you detect and compensate for possible omissions and inadequacies in your review materials.

BEHAVIOR I PRACTICE TEST

ANSWER SHEET

	ANS	CON
1.		
2.		
3.		
4.		
5.		
6.		
7.		
8.		
9.		
10.		
11.		
12.		
13.		

	ANS	CON
14.		
15.		
16.		
17.		
18.		
19.		
20.		
21.		
22.		
23.		
24.		
25.		

SEE PAGE 25 FOR INSTRUCTIONS
SEE PAGE 211 FOR ANSWERS

CUT HERE

STUDY SUGGESTION

Can you draw the profile side of an American penny from memory? Return to Chapter 2 for some advice on memory and how to avoid equating familiarity with adequate knowledge.

BEHAVIOR I

1. The pituitary secretion of endorphins is closely lined to the secretion of adrenocorticotropic hormone(ACTH) so that endorphins facilitate the ability to respond to
(A) retarded growth
(B) severe hypertension
(C) stress
(D) chronic pain
(E) tachycardia

2. Consumption of alcohol is associated with all the following EXCEPT
(A) inhibition of mobility of macrophages
(B) inhibition of proliferation of T cells
(C) inhibition of cytotoxicity of T cells
(D) inhibition of production of antibodies
(E) damage to the thymus

3. The transmitter that ultimately mediates all overt behavior is:
(A) Dopamine
(B) Dopamine-B-hydroxylase
(C) 6-Hydroxydopamine
(D) Norepinephrine
(E) Acetylcholine

4. The substance produced by smoking behavior which contributes to increased prevalence of fatal and nonfatalcardiovascular disease:
(A) Nicotine
(B) Carbon monoxide
(C) Hydrogen cyanide
(D) Both hydrogen cyanide and carbon monoxide
(E) Both nicotine and carbon monoxide

5. The most important (frequent) genetic cause of mental retardation is
(A) Bartholin-Patau syndrome
(B) Edwards' syndrome
(C) Down's syndrome
(D) Turner's syndrome
(E) Klinefelter's syndrome

6. A disorder resulting from a single gene defect that may produce severe mental problems is
(A) manic-depressive psychosis
(B) dyslexia
(C) phenylketonuria
(D) Porter's syndrome
(E) Down's syndrome

7. Although there is no uniform asthmatic personality type, the most frequent psychological characteristic of boys with bronchial asthma is
(A) hostility
(B) general anxiety
(C) frustrated oral needs
(D) dependency
(E) latent homosexuality

8. In the assessment of personality, the normative and objective method refers to
(A) the use of "inkblot" techniques
(B) sophisticated techniques for measuring the accuracy of a person's perception of reality
(C) predictions of behavior on the basis of intensive interviewing
(D) predictions of behavior on the basis of data from personality tests
(E) a way of really evaluating personality rather than of simply assessing how a person behaves

9. Erik Erikson's theory of the life cycle and growth of the ego is reflected in which of the following statements?

(A) Sexual drive is crucial in determining the sense of identity

(B) Ego maturation is genetically predetermined; cultural influences are of minor importance

(C) There are eight stages characterized by crises whose satisfactory resolution is essential to the development of a healthy sense of identity

(D) The phases of development are characterized in turn by aggressive, affiliative, achievement, nurturance, and power motives

(E) People are burdened with too many ego functions; society would benefit from stricter and more economic processes of socialization

10. Which are the two main functions of the family in America?

(A) Socialization of children and nurturance and security of adult personalities

(B) Achievement of economic security and regulation of sexual behavior

(C) Socialization of children and regulation of sexual behavior

(D) Achievement of economic security and perpetuation of lines of inheritance

(E) Perpetuation of lines of inheritance and stabilization of adult personalities

11. All the following factors are included in gender identity EXCEPT

(A) gender role behavior

(B) parental and cultural attitudes

(C) external genitalia

(D) sexual behavior

(E) genetic influence

12. The intervention style that is most effective in relieving the stress of surgery and enhancing the outcome is to provide the patient with

(A) problem-focused information

(B) emotion-focused information

(C) a match between personality factors and treatment style

(D) maximum family support

(E) as much preparatory medical information as can be understood

13. Stroking one's own hair, rearranging clothing, pushing hair away from one's face is body language behavior that may be interpreted as:

(A) Not willing to enter into a communicative interaction

(B) Angry, hostile, or upset

(C) "I'm interested in you. Notice me."

(D) Assertive and domineering

(E) Submissive and fearful

14. The view that leadership is a reciprocal process of social influence with leaders and followers being influenced by each other is known as

(A) situational leadership

(B) contingency model

(C) social facilitation

(D) collective behavior model

(E) transactional leadership

15. The learning mechanism that pairs a neutral stimulus with a stimulus that produces a known response until the neutral stimulus alone produces the known response:

(A) Contact desensitization

(B) Shaping

(C) Systematic desensitization

(D) Operant conditioning

(E) Classical conditioning

16. The Hawthorne effect is best illustrated by which of the following situations?

(A) Of a group of factory workers who volunteer for a study of productivity and piecework payment, more than 80 percent quit the project because of the influence of nonvolunteer workers

(B) A group of factory workers who volunteer for such a study demonstrate an improvement in work rate greater than that associated with changed working conditions because they feel specially treated

(C) Work rate increases when workers are allowed frequent brief rest periods

(D) Productivity increases when workers have more opportunity to participate in the organization of their daily routine

(E) Although many workers initially are reluctant to have their routines changed and are suspicious of managerial motives, such changes are quickly accepted if their connection with improved working conditions is demonstrated

17. The percentage of married women who were employed rose from 5.5 percent in 1900 to what percentage in 1978?

(A) 21 percent

(B) 31 percent

(C) 41 percent

(D) 51 percent

(E) 61 percent

18. The risk for hypertension is greatest among

(A) whites of lower socioeconomic status

(B) blacks of lower socioeconomic status

(C) whites of higher socioeconomic status

(D) blacks of higher socioeconomic status

(E) upwardly mobile middle-class whites

19. All the following statements about persons of lower socioeconomic status and attitudes toward health are true EXCEPT

(A) their medical needs are greater

(B) they are less concerned about their health

(C) they have a chronically low utilization rate of health services

(D) their health-seeking behaviors do not change even when financial barriers are removed

(E) they are more alienated from society and medical institutions

20. All the following statements about hyperthyroidism are true EXCEPT that it

(A) may be the cause of frank psychosis

(B) is more frequent in women than in men

(C) may be precipitated by acute emotional stress

(D) is associated with mental retardation in children

(E) is associated with tension and hyperexcitability

21. The leading cause of death in the elderly(65 and older) is

(A) cancer

(B) cerebrovascular disease(stroke)

(C) suicide

(D) heart disease

(E) chronic obstructive pulmonary disease

22. Human immunodeficiency virus(HIV) is spread primarily by all the following EXCEPT

(A) exchange of bodily fluids during sex

(B) sharing of needles or other drug paraphernalia

(C) blood transfusion

(D) fomites contaminated by respiratory infection

(E) perinatal contact of an infected mother with her infant

23. All the following statements about obesity are true EXCEPT

(A) obesity increases the risk of developing diabetes approximately fourfold

(B) obese persons are more likely to die in automobile accidents than are members of the population in general

(C) obesity increases the severity of most health problems

(D) obesity is the leading cause of hypertension

(E) obesity has been linked to complications from surgery and infections

24. Select the disease which is associated with an approximate 3 percent in mortality between 1970 and 1986:

(A) Disease of the heart

(B) Malignant neoplasm

(C) Chronic obstructive pulmonary disease

(D) Cerebrovascular disease

(E) None of the above

25. The revised third edition of the Diagnostic and Statistical Manual of Mental Disorders(DSM III-R) offers an improvement over earlier psychiatric classifications. Its major advantage is that it

(A) identifies mental illness as a disease

(B) deals with predisposing factors

(C) confirms and supports the nosological system

(D) is an all-inclusive classification system

(E) is a multiaxial classification system

BEHAVIOR II PRACTICE TEST
ANSWER SHEET

CUT HERE

	ANS	CON
1.		
2.		
3.		
4.		
5.		
6.		
7.		
8.		
9.		
10.		
11.		
12.		
13.		

	ANS	CON
14.		
15.		
16.		
17.		
18.		
19.		
20.		
21.		
22.		
23.		
24.		
25.		

SEE PAGE **25** FOR INSTRUCTIONS
SEE PAGE **212** FOR ANSWERS

STUDY SUGGESTION

Which option(s) in the question below can be ruled out even without seeing the photomicrograph that should accompany this question? (See answer at bottom of page 56.)

A perimenopausal woman complains of slight difficulty swallowing, fatigue and a change in bowel habits. The photomicrograph is of her thyroid gland. This disorder is

A. Subacute thyroiditis   B. Thyrotoxicosis
C. Autoimmune thyroiditis   D. Conversion hysteria
E. Riedel's thyroiditis

BEHAVIOR II

1. When persons with a type A pattern of coronary-prone behavior are subjected to stressful situations, they exhibit increases in all the following EXCEPT

(A) plasma norepinephrine

(B) systolic blood pressure

(C) heart rate

(D) occipital alpha activity

(E) cortisol

2. The gate control theory of pain assumes all the following EXCEPT that

(A) the substantia gelatinosa is the primary vehicle for gating

(B) the spinal gate mechanism is influenced by nerve impulses that descend from the brain

(C) the activity in the large nerve fibers will tend to facilitate the transmission by opening the gate

(D) motivation, emotion, and cognition modulate the pain experience

(E) the spinal gate mechanism in the dorsal horn modulates the transmission from afferent fibers to spinal cord transmission cells

3. A decline in heart rate, blood pressure, and respiration and increase in gastrointestinal movements suggests which stage of sleep.

(A) Stage I REM sleep

(B) Stage 1 NREM sleep

(C) Stages I through 4 slow wave sleep (NREM)

(D) Stage 4 delta wave sleep (NREM)

(E) Stage 2 NREM sleep

4. Heredity accounts for approximately what percentage of total variation in IQ scores within a family?

(A) 5 percent

(B) 25 percent

(C) 50 percent

(D) 75 percent

(E) 100 percent

5. The complex of severe psychologic disorders known as schizophrenia has a demonstrable basis that is characterized as

(A) environmentally determined

(B) polygenic

(C) a chromosomal aberration

(D) a simple recessive trait

(E) an inborn error of metabolism

6. According to psychoanalytic theory, which of the following statements about the development of the superego is true?

(A) It is present at birth

(B) It begins to develop during the first 2 years of life

(C) It begins to develop during the fifth or sixth year of life

(D) It begins to develop during puberty

(E) It begins to develop in late adolescence

7. Anterograde amnesia is associated with which of the following disorders?

(A) Mild retardation

(B) Hypochondriasis

(C) Sociopathy

(D) Korsakoff's psychosis

(E) Manic-depressive psychosis

8. In operant conditioning, the rate of extinction is most effectively slowed when the response or learning has been maintained on a reinforcement schedule of

(A) fixed ratio

(B) variable ratio

(C) fixed interval reinforcement

(D) continuous reinforcement

(E) piecework reinforcement

9. Nutritional experts have recommended all the following behavioral tips for weight control EXCEPT

(A) eating slowly

(B) taking small portions of food

(C) waiting 20 minutes before taking a second helping

(D) watching television or reading while you are eating

(E) recording all food intake in a "dietary diary"

10. The environmental factor with the most underused potential for developing cognitive and interpersonal competence in children is the

(A) school

(B) family setting

(C) community mental health center

(D) health care system

(E) child welfare agency

11. The World Health Organization has stated that the most serious worldwide drug problem is

(A) cocaine

(B) alcohol

(C) marijuana

(D) amphetamines

(E) opium

12. All the following statements about prenatal and perinatal development are true EXCEPT that

(A) the developmental consequences of prematurity are resolved within the first 18 months

(B) prematurity is more frequent in mothers from lower socioeconomic groups

(C) maternal anxiety is associated with incidence of colic in the neonate

(D) marital conflict during pregnancy may affect the quality of early mother- child interaction

(E) the incidence of neonatal retardation is highest in mothers who are less than 20 or more than 35 years of age

13. Interpersonal relationship studies have concluded that the most critical element to assure compliance behavior in a physician-patient relationship is

(A) the exchange of accurate information and facts

(B) the congruence of expectations of physician and patient

(C) similarity of physician's and patient's age

(D) recognition and down-playing of social class differences between physician and patient

(E) allowing for the patient to be rewarded in some way for compliance

14. Which of the following is the leading consumer of health care dollars?

(A) Cardiovascular disease

(B) Cancer

(C) Gastrointestinal disease

(D) Respiratory disease

(E) Accidents

15. According to the Yale studies of attitude change, communicators can increase their persuasiveness by

(A) discussing only one side of an issue when an audience is hostile

(B) presenting only one side of an issue when a competing persuader will get a chance to present the other side

(C) discussing one side of the argument when it is not important to achieve long-lasting attitude change

(D) de-emphasizing their own expertise

(E) allowing an audience of limited intelligence to draw its own conclusions

16. In the study of group behavior, deindividuation has been found to produce all the following effects EXCEPT

(A) weakened restraints against impulsive behavior

(B) inability to monitor or regulate one's own behavior

(C) decreased sensitivity to immediate cues

(D) lessened concern about evaluations by others

(E) lowered ability to engage in rational planning

17. Obesity has been well documented as a primary contributing factor in the development of each of the following diseases EXCEPT

(A) adult-onset diabetes

(B) hypertension

(C) gallbladder disease

(D) arthritis

(E) myocardial hypertrophy

18. All the following statements about child abuse are true EXCEPT

(A) fathers abuse their children more often than do mothers

(B) child-abusing parents often were abused by their own parents

(C) prematurely born children are more often abused than are normal-term children

(D) parents are more likely to abuse one "scapegoat" child than to abuse all their children

(E) younger children are more often abused than are older children

19. An effective strategy for maintaining a strong relationship between employee performance and employee satisfaction is to

(A) give all employees equal raises

(B) pay all employees what they are worth in the marketplace

(C) pay all employees more than they are worth in the marketplace

(D) pay good performers much more than poor performers

(E) pay good performers slightly more than poor performers

20. Essential hypertension has been frequently associated with all the following EXCEPT

(A) repressed anger

(B) acutely stressful events

(C) familial history of hypertension

(D) decreased sympathetic nervous system activity

(E) decreased parasympathetic inhibition

21. Empirical findings about patterns of disease and illness include all the following EXCEPT

(A) a large range of symptoms, e.g., headache, upset stomach, and sore muscles, is found in the general population on any given day

(B) a very small percentage of persons experiencing symptoms of disease or illness seeks medical care

(C) individual persons show highly diverse reactions to the presence of many disease symptoms

(D) it is important for physicians to understand how patients interpret their perceived physical signs and symptoms

(E) persons are relatively independent of communication from others in deciding on the meaning of their own unexpected physiological changes

22. The single most significant source of preventable morbidity and premature mortality is

(A) environmental pollution
(B) crime and homicide
(C) auto and home accidents
(D) poor nutrition
(E) cigarette smoking

23. Select the health care payment plan which it is most closely associated with a compulsory hospital insurance plan whose cost is shared by employees and employers through Social Security payroll taxes

(A) Medicare
(B) National Health Insurance
(C) Medicaid
(D) Blue Cross
(E) Blue Shield

24. Which of the following statements best describes the Likert technique of attitude measurement?

(A) Subjects indicate on five-point scales the extent of their agreement with a set of attitude statements

(B) Subjects indicate whether they agree with each of a series of attitude statements, which are equally spaced along an attitude continuum

(C) Subjects' responses to an open-ended interview are coded by content analysis

(D) Subjects judge a particular concept on a series of bipolar semantic scales

(E) Subjects check all acceptable items in a set of statements arranged in order of "difficulty of acceptance"

25. Two drugs were administered in several different doses, and the effects were measured and recorded. The data were subjected to regression and correlation analyses. The computed regression lines and correlation coefficients are presented below. Which of the following statements is true?

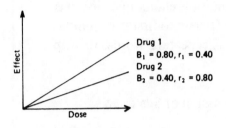

Drug 1
$B_1 = 0.80$, $r_1 = 0.40$
Drug 2
$B_2 = 0.40$, $r_2 = 0.80$

(A) In general, the strength of the causal relationship between two variables is indicated by the square of the correlation coefficient

(B) The proportion of variation in response to Drug 1 accounted for by dose is $(0.80)^2$

(C) The data indicate Drug 1 is more effective than Drug 2

(D) The data indicate Drug 1 is more potent than Drug 2

(E) There is more variability in responses to Drug 1 than to Drug 2

STUDY SUGGESTION

True or False:
When approaching a multiple choice question, it is most productive and efficient to first use elimination strategies, such as repeating words, to help focus your thinking.

See page 58 for a discussion of this issue.

**ANSWER TO THE QUESTION
ON PAGE 50**

1. Option D (conversion hysteria is a "ridiculous option" and can be ruled out.

2. Option B (Thyrotoxicosis) is less likely than Options A, C, and E since the word Thyroiditis repeats in those alternatives.

3. The correct answer is C.

BIOCHEMISTRY I PRACTICE TEST

ANSWER SHEET

	ANS	CON			ANS	CON
1.				**14.**		
2.				**15.**		
3.				**16.**		
4.				**17.**		
5.				**18.**		
6.				**19.**		
7.				**20.**		
8.				**21.**		
9.				**22.**		
10.				**23.**		
11.				**24.**		
12.				**25.**		
13.						

CUT HERE

SEE PAGE **25** FOR INSTRUCTIONS
SEE PAGE **212** FOR ANSWERS

STUDY SUGGESTION

When answering questions, never use elimination strategies until after you have applied all of your knowledge and deductive reasoning skills (see Chapter 8).

Consider the issue on page 56. The statement is False.

BIOCHEMISTRY I

1. Which of the following amino acids is ketogenic but not glucogenic?

(A) Isoleucine

(B) Tyrosine

(C) Leucine

(D) Phenylalanine

(E) Threonine

2. A purely competitive enzyme inhibitor has which of the following kinetic effects?

(A) Increases Km without affecting Vmax

(B) Decreases Km with affecting Vmax

(C) Increases Vmax without affecting Km

(D) Decreases Vmax without affecting Km

(E) Decreases both Vmax and Km

3. The approximate isoelectric pH (pHl) for aspartic acid (pKαl = 2.09, pKα2 = 3.86, pKα3 = 9.82) is represented by which of the following values?

(A) 2.09

(B) 2.97

(C) 3.86

(D) 6.84

(E) 9.82

4. The formation of thymine dimers as a result of sunburn

(A) requires an enzyme repair mechanism that utilizes ligase

(B) does not affect pyrimidines

(C) creates covalent bonds between thymines on opposite nucleotide strands

(D) is transcribed as frameshift mutations

(E) is repaired by thymidine hydroxylase

5. In humans all the following amino acids are nonessential EXCEPT

(A) arginine

(B) tyrosine

(C) proline

(D) valine

(E) cysteine

6. For thiol protease, select the most appropriate class of enzyme.

(A) Chymotrypsin

(B) Pancreozymin

(C) Papain

(D) Carboxpeptidase A

(E) Pepsin

7. Some of the enzymes utilized in DNA replication are (1) DNA-directed DNA polymerase, (2) unwinding proteins, (3) DNA polymerase I, (4) DNA-directed RNA polymerase, and (5) DNA ligase. What is the correct sequence of their use during DNA synthesis?

(A) 4,3,1,2,5

(B) 2,3,4,1,5

(C) 4,2,1,5,3

(D) 4,2,1,3,5

(E) 2,4,1,3,5

8. Modification of mRNA so that a signal sequence is added to the amino terminus of the cytosolic protein, a-globin, results in

(A) no change in physiology of the protein

(B) proteolytic cleavage within the cytosol

(C) translocation across the endoplasmic reticulum

(D) cytosolic localization of the protein

(E) signal recognition particle synthesis

9. Tetracycline prevents synthesis of polypeptides by

(A) competing with MRNA for ribosomal binding sites

(B) blocking mRNA formation from DNA

(C) releasing peptides from MRNA-tRNA complexes

(D) inhibiting TRNA binding to mRNA

(E) preventing amino acid binding by tRNA

10. Carbamoyl phosphate synthetase functioning in cytosol, but not mitochondria,

(A) is inhibited by uridine triphosphate

(B) is activated by acetyglutamate

(C) has a high activity

(D) cannot be found in liver

(E) is involved in purine biosynthesis

11. Which compound.inhibits transcription by locking the first phosphodiester bond in the presumptive RNA chain

(A) Streptomycin

(B) Rifamycin B

(C) Tetracycline

(D) Actinomycin D

(E) None of the above

12. All the following statements about mammalian energy metabolism are true EXCEPT

(A) ATP is formed in the absence of O_2

(B) ATP hydrolysis is an exergonic reaction

(C) ATP is formed in the presence of O_2

(D) heat produced by ATP hydrolysis specifically drives other reactions

(E) NADH can be utilized for form ATP

13. All the following statements about glycogen metabolism are true EXCEPT that

(A) cyclic AMP-activated protein kinase stimulates glycogen synthase

(B) phosphorylase kinase is activated by phosphorylation

(C) phosphorylase b is activated by phosphorylation

(D) cyclic AMP levels are raised by epinephrine and glucagon stimulation of adenylate cyclase

(E) a futile cycle of glycogenesis and glycogenolysis is prevented by second-messenger regulation

14. Which of the following occurs in nonshivering thermogenesis?

(A) Glucose is oxidized to lactate

(B) Fatty acids uncouple oxidative phosphorylation

(C) Ethanol is formed

(D) ATP is burned for heat production

(E) Adipose tissue is functionally absent

15. Which of the following is noted in Cushing's syndrome, a tumor-associated disease of the adrenal cortex?

(A) Decreased production of epinephrine

(B) Excessive production of epinephrine

(C) Excessive production of vasopressin

(D) Excessive production of cortisol

(E) Decreased production of cortisol

16. All the following compounds are members of the electron transport chain EXCEPT

(A) ubiquinone (coenzyme Q)

(B) cytochrome c

(C) nicotinamide adenine dinucleotide (NAD)

(D) flavin adenine dinucleotide (FAD)

(E) carnitine

17. Studies of the action of two anti-coagulants - dicumarol and warfarin (the latter also a hemorrhagic rat poison) -have revealed that

(A) vitamin C is necessary for the synthesis of fibrinogen

(B) vitamin C activates fibrinogen

(C) vitamin K is a clotting factor

(D) vitamin K is essential for y carboxylation of glutamate

(E) the action of vitamin E is antago-nized by these compounds

18. The activated group or unit with which uridine diphosphate (UDP) is most closely associated is

(A) Electrons

(B) Phosphoryl

(C) Acyl

(D) Aldehyde

(E) Glucose

19. ATP is the direct source of free energy in all the following active transport systems of mammals EXCEPT

(A) NA$^+$ - K

(B) glucose

(C) Ca^{2+}

(D) H$^+$ of stomach

(E) proton pump of endocytic vesicles

20. The oxygen dissociation curve for meoglobin is shifted to the right by

(A) decreased 0_2 tension

(B) decreased CO_2 tension

(C) increased CO_2 tension

(D) increased N_2 tension

(E) increased pH

21. All the following descriptions of calcium are correct EXCEPT

(A) it diffuses as a divalent cation

(B) it is required as a cofactor for many reactions

(C) it freely diffuses across the endoplasmic reticulum of muscle cells

(D) it is most highly concentrated in bone

(E) it is excreted through the intestinal limen

22. Most major metabolic pathways are considered to be either mainly anabolic or catabolic.Which of the following pathways is most correctly considered to be amphibolic?

(A) Lipolysis

(B) Glycolysis

(C) β-Oxidation of fatty acids

(D) Citric acid cycle

(E) Gluconeogenesis

23. The normal blood concentration of urea is

(A) 25 mg/dl plasma

(B) 80 mg/dl plasma

(C) 3.5 g/dl plasma

(D) 15 g/dl blood

(E) 50 g/dl blood

24. Analysis of pH 8.6 electrophoretic patterns of hemoglobin isolated from the blood of patients heterzygous for the sickle cell gene would reveal

(A) one band
(B) two bands
(C) three bands
(D) four bands
(E) five bands

25. When proteins denatured in sodium dodecyl sulfate (SDS) and mercaptoethanol are separated by electrophoresis,

(A) the denatured proteins have a large net negative charge
(B) cations of SDS bind to the protein
(C) disulfide bridges are maintained
(D) the direction of electrophoretic movement is positive to negative
(E) the native protein charge is significant

BIOCHEMISTRY II PRACTICE TEST

ANSWER SHEET

	ANS	CON
1.		
2.		
3.		
4.		
5.		
6.		
7.		
8.		
9.		
10.		
11.		
12.		
13.		

	ANS	CON
14.		
15.		
16.		
17.		
18.		
19.		
20.		
21.		
22.		
23.		
24.		
25.		

SEE PAGE **25** FOR INSTRUCTIONS
SEE PAGE **212** FOR ANSWERS

CUT HERE

STUDY SUGGESTION

True or False:
When approaching a multiple choice exam, it is most productive and efficient to skip the difficult questions, leaving them blank, until all easier questions have been answered.

See page 70 for a discussion of this issue.

BIOCHEMISTRY II

1. Analysis of pH 8.6 electrophoretic patterns of hemoglobin isolated from the blood of patients heterozygous for the sickle cell gene would reveal

(A) one band

(B) two bands

(C) three bands

(D) four bands

(E) five bands

2. When proteins denatured in sodium dodecyl sulfate (SDS) and mercaptoethanol are separated by electrophoresis,

(A) the denatured proteins have a large net negative charge

(B) cations of SDS bind to the protein

(C) disulfide bridges are maintained

(D) the direction of electrophoretic movement is positive to negative

(E) the native protein charge is significant

3. All the following statements concerning immunoglobulins are true EXCEPT

(A) the distinctiveness of the heavy chains gives the different classes of immunoglobulins their unique biological characteristics

(B) IgG is the principle antibody in the serum

(C) the light chains are similar in each class of immunoglobulin

(D) the constant regions of the heavy chains are the same in each class of immunoglobulin

(E) IgA is the major immunoglobulin found in external secretions

4. If curve X in the graph shown below represents no inhibition for the reaction of some enzyme with its substrate, which of the other curves would represent competitive inhibition of the same reaction?

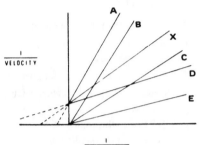

(A) A

(B) B

(C) C

(D) D

(E) E

5. All the following statements correctly describe insulin EXCEPT

(A) it is thought to be an anabolic signal to cells that glucose is abundant

(B) it is converted from proinsulin to insulin primarily following secretion from b cells

(C) it is inactive when in the proinsulin form

(D) it is a small polypeptide composed of two chains connected by disulfide bridges

(E) its action is antagonistic to that of glucagon

6. For the familial disorder, Phenylk-etonuria (PKU), select the compound that accumulates in the urine.

(A) Tryptophan

(B) Homocysteine

(C) Dopa

(D) Phenylpyruvate

(E) Keto acids

7. Which of the following mutations is most likely to be lethal?

(A) Substitution of adenine for cytosine

(B) Substitution of cytosine for guanine

(C) Substitution of methylcytosine for cytosine

(D) Deletion of three nucleotides

(E) Insertion of one nucleotide

8. The function of signal recognition particles is to

(A) cleave signal sequences

(B) detect cytosolic proteins

(C) direct the signal sequence to ribosomes

(D) bind ribosomes to endoplasmic reticulum

(E) bind mRNA to ribosomes

9. Chronic alcoholics require more ethanol than do nondrinkers to become intoxicated because of a higher level of specific enzyme. However, independent of specific enzyme levels, the availability of what other substance is rate-limiting in the clearance of ethanol?

(A) NADH

(B) NAD⁺

(C) FADH

(D) FAD⁺

(E) NADPH

10. Which one of the following single-stranded DNA molecules would be palindromic in the double-stranded state?

(A) A-T-G-C-C-G-T-A

(B) A-T-G-C-T-A-C-G

(C) G-T-C-A-T-G-A-C

(D) G-T-A-T-C-T-A-T

(E) G-C-T-A-T-G-A-C

11. Select the reaction that the enzyme, b DNA polymerase catalyzes.

(A) Initiation of *E. coli* DNA synthesis

(B) Replication of DNA

(C) Repair of DNA lesions

(D) Joining of the ends of DNA

(E) None of the above

12. Chylomicra, intermediate-density lipoproteins (IDL), low-density lipoproteins (LDL), and very low-density lipoproteins (VLDL) all are serum lipoproteins. What is the correct ordering of these particles from the lowest to the greatest density?

(A) LDL > IDL > VLDL > chylomicra

(B) Chylomicra > VLDL > IDL>LDL

(C) VLDL > IDL > LDL > chylomicra

(D) Chylomicra > IDL > VLDL > LDL

(E) LDL > VLDL > IDL > chylomicra

13. After a well-rounded breakfast, all the following would be expected to occur EXCEPT

(A) decreased activity of pyruvate carboxylase

(B) increased activity of acetyl CoA carboxylase

(C) increased rate of glycogenolysis

(D) increased rate of protein synthesis

(E) decreased activity of phosphoenol-pyruvate carboxykinase

14. The nascent 5' end of transcribed eukaryotic mRNA is quickly modified to contain

(A) 7-methylguanylate

(B) 6-dimethyladenine

(C) polyuridine

(D) pseudouridine

(E) polyadenylate

15. In the generalized synthetic pathway below, what do NuDP and X stand for, respectively?

NuDP sugars + NuDP sugar amines
    + glucose-ceramide → → X

(A) UDP and ganglioside

(B) UDP and sphingomyelin

(C) CDP and sphingomyelin

(D) CDP and glucocerebroside

(E) ADP and ganglioside

16. Increased reabsorption of water from the kidney is the major consequence of which of the following hormones?

(A) Cortisol

(B) Insulin

(C) Vasopressin

(D) Glucagon

(E) Aldosterone

17. Which statement is true concerning folic acid?

(A) It links to the e-amino group of lysine residues of enzymes

(B) It derives a nitrogen from *p*-aminobenzoic acid

(C) It functions by making and breaking its own disulfide bond

(D) It is a synonym for vitamin B_1

(E) It is a cofactor in deamination of amino acids

18. All the following statements apply to the Pasteur effect EXCEPT that

(A) under aerobic conditions, adenosine triphosphate (ATP) causes allosteric inhibition of phosphofructokinase

(B) under anaerobic conditions, 18 times as much glucose per cell is utilized to generate the equivalent amount of ATP than would be generated aerobically

(C) lactate accumulation becomes quantitative under conditions when oxygen becomes freely available

(D) allosteric inhibition of phosphofructokinase by citrate occurs under aerobic conditions

(E) glucose utilization decreases greatly under aerobic conditions

19. In order for a reconstituted system of myosin-coated beads to show structured movement in vitro, the appropriate medium must contain ATP and at least

(A) calcium + actin

(B) calcium + actin + tropomyosin

(C) calcium + actin + tropomyosin + troponin

(D) actin + tropomyosin + troponin + microtubules

(E) tropomyosin + troponin

20. Which of the following enzymes or enzyme systems is localized in the inner membrane of the mitochondrion?

(A) Acyl CoA synthetases

(B) Isocitrate dehydrogenase

(C) Fatty acyl CoA oxidation enzymes

(D) Succinate dehydrogenase

(E) Nucleoside diphosphate kinase

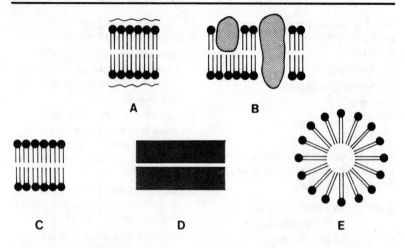

21. Which of the diagrammatic structures shown above most clearly represents a model of the configuration that lipids are expected to take following emulsification by bile during the intestinal digestive process?

(A) A

(B) B

(C) C

(D) D

(E) E

22. Sugar residues commonly found in glycoproteins include all the following EXCEPT

(A) fructose

(B) galactose

(C) sialic acid

(D) mannose

(E) N-acetylglucosamine

23. During a normal fast between meals, blood glucose levels are maintained by all the following EXCEPT

(A) utilization of fatty acids by skeletal muscle

(B) utilization of fatty acids by liver

(C) utilization of ketone bodies by brain

(D) glycogenolysis in liver

(E) lipolysis in adipose tissue

24. Glucose may be oxidized by all of the following EXCEPT

(A) liver

(B) brain

(C) heart

(D) erythrocytes

(E) skeletal muscle

25. All the following contain an iron porphyrin EXCEPT

(A) catalase

(B) hemoglobin

(C) NADH dehydrogenase

(D) myoglobin

(E) cytochrome *c*

GENETICS PRACTICE TEST

ANSWER SHEET

	ANS	CON
1.		
2.		
3.		
4.		
5.		
6.		
7.		
8.		
9.		
10.		
11.		
12.		
13.		

	ANS	CON
14.		
15.		
16.		
17.		
18.		
19.		
20.		
21.		
22.		
23.		
24.		
25.		

SEE PAGE **25** FOR INSTRUCTIONS
SEE PAGE **213** FOR ANSWERS

CUT HERE

STUDY SUGGESTION

Never leave blanks as you take an exam to ensure that you
   –get the benefit of first hunches
   –don't waste time re-reading questions
   –don't leave blanks and lose points
   –don't make transcription errors

Consider the issue on page 64. The statement is False.

GENETICS

1. Chromosomal imbalance is most frequent during the following stage of human development

(A) embryonic

(B) fetal

(C) neonatal

(D) childhood

(E) adult

2. Clinical indication for karyotyping include all of the following EXCEPT

(A) multiple malformations in a newborn

(B) single malformation in a newborn

(C) mental retardation of unknown etiology

(D) offspring with chromosomal rearrangement

(E) recurrent pregnancy loss

3. - 7. The major blood group locus in humans produces types A (genotypes AA or AO), B (genotypes BB or BO), AB (genotype AB), or O (genotype OO). Which children might be offspring of the following parents.

(A) Type AB child

(B) Type B child

(C) Type O child

(D) All of above

(E) None of above

3. Type A father, Type O mother

4. Type O father, Type AB mother

5. Type AB father, Type O mother

6. Type A father, Type B mother

7. Type A mother, Type A father

8. - 10. A baby boy dies in the newborn period with severe hyperammonemia. Prior his death, he is diagnosed as having OTC (ornithine transcarbamyolase) deficiency. OTC deficiency is an X-linked disorder of urea cycle metabolism which, in its classic form, is lethal in males. Answer the following questions with regard to the family.

8. The likelihood that the proband's disease is the result of a new mutation is:

(A) 100%

(B) 67%

(C) 50%

(D) 33%

(E) 25%

9. Subsequent testing reveals that the proband's mother is a carrier of the disease. The chance that her next child will be affected is:

(A) 67%

(B) 50%

(C) 33%

(D) 25%

(E) 0%

10. The proband's mother remarries. The chance that her next child will be affected is

(A) 67%

(B) 50%

(C) 33%

(D) 25%

(E) 0%

11. Of the following karyotypes, which would not be expected from meiotic segregation of a 46,XX,t (14q21q) Robertsonian translocation? Assume union with normal gametes to produce the zygotes.

(A) Monosomy 21

(B) Trisomy 21

(C) 45,XY,t (14q21q)

(D) 46,XX

(E) 46,XX,-21,+t (144q21q)

12. - 16. Match the following numbered terms with their partial definitions

(A) One lesion, serial consequences for related embryonic structures

(B) Abnormality extrinsic to structure, i.e. decreased perfusion because of vascular blow-out or amniotic band

(C) Abnormality extrinsic to structure, i.e. crowding because of uterine fibroid tumor of oligohydramnios (scanty amniotic fluid)

(D) Abnormality intrinsic to structure, i.e. horseshoe kidney

(E) One lesion, multiple anomalies affecting unrelated embryonic structures

12. Syndrome

13. Sequence

14. Disruption

15. Deformation

16. Malformation

17. - 21. Match the following (numbered) with the appropriate ribonucleic acid (lettered)

(A) mRNA

(B) DNA

(C) tRNA

(D) rRNA

17. 3' ACCTG 5'

18. Contained in ribosomes

19. approximately 80 nucleotides long

20. forms a template for the synthesis of polypeptide chains

21. double stranded

22. - 24. Match the following partial definition with its partial definition

(A) Conversion of triplet codons into amino acids

(B) Duplication of DNA

(C) Pairing of complimentary strands of nucleic acids

(D) Conversion of DNA to RNA

22. Replication

23. Translation

24. Hybridization

25. The most common type of mutation found in DNA is

(A) Insertion

(B) Gene deletion

(C) Small intragenic deletion

(D) Point mutation

MICROBIOLOGY I PRACTICE TEST

ANSWER SHEET

CUT HERE

	ANS	CON
1.		
2.		
3.		
4.		
5.		
6.		
7.		
8.		
9.		
10.		
11.		
12.		
13.		

	ANS	CON
14.		
15.		
16.		
17.		
18.		
19.		
20.		
21.		
22.		
23.		
24.		
25.		

SEE PAGE 25 FOR INSTRUCTIONS
SEE PAGE 213 FOR ANSWERS

STUDY SUGGESTION

True or False:
When approaching a multiple-choice exam, it is most productive and efficient to become concerned and speed up if several questions in a row take longer than 55 seconds.

See page 80 for a discussion of this issue.

MICROBIOLOGY I

1. A patient presents with a request for testing for human immunodeficiency virus (HIV) because of a weekend fling of promiscuous sexual activity 2 weeks ago. Given that time frame of possible infection, what is the best, most cost-efficient test to order?

(A) HIV enzyme immunoassay (EIA) for antibody

(B) HIV EIA for antigen

(C) HIV western blot

(D) Polymerase chain reaction (PCR) for HIV

(E) HIV culture

2. A hospital patient received 3 units of whole blood and developed severe hepatitis 8 weeks later. The most probable cause of that hepatitis is

(A) hepatitis A virus

(B) hepatitis B virus

(C) hepatitis D (delta) virus

(D) non-A, non-B hepatitis (hepatitis C) virus

(E) cytomegalovirus

3. Since commercially prepared HTLV-I enzyme immunoassay was licensed by the FDA, blood units in the U.S. have been screened for HTLV-I prior to release. This testing would be necessary in all the following components EXCEPT

(A) plasma

(B) whole blood

(C) red blood cells

(D) platelets

(E) white blood cells

4. Infection with Epstein-Barr virus (EBV) results in the development of virus-specific antibodies. In the case of infectious mononucleosis, for the antibody, EBNA-Ab, choose the description with which it is most likely to be associated.

(A) Appears 2 weeks to several months after onset and is present more often in atypical cases of infectious mononucleosis

(B) Appears 3 to 4 weeks after onset; titers correlate with severity of clinical illness

(C) Arises early in the course of the illness; detectable titers persist a lifetime

(D) Appears late in the course of the disease and persists a lifetime

(E) Arises early in the course of the illness, and then titers fall rapidly

5. Choose the description most likely to be associated with hepatitis, HBeAg.

(A) Is usually the first viral marker detected in blood after HBV infection

(B) May be the only detectable serologic marker during the early convalescent phase of an HBV infection ("window phase")

(C) Appears in the blood soon after infection, rises to very high concentrations, and falls rapidly with the onset of hepathic disease

(D) Found within the nuclei of infected hepatocytes and not generally in the peripheral circulation

(E) Closely associated with hepatitis B infectivity and DNA polymerase activity

6. An antral biopsy was performed on a patient with symptoms of gastric ulcers. A Giemsa stain of the tissue revealed curved, rod-shaped bacteria. Culture on enriched chocolate agar, inactivated at 35° C, revealed a gram-negative, comma-shaped bacillus. The most likely identification is

(A) *Campylobacter jejuni*

(B) *Campylobacter (Helicobacter) pylori*

(C) *Vibria cholerae*

(D) *Mycobacterium*

(E) *Escherichia coli*

7. Bacteria cause disease in a number of ways. One mechanism of pathogenesis is the secretion of potent protein toxins. All the following diseases are caused by microbial protein toxins EXCEPT

(A) tetanus

(B) botulism

(C) Shigella dysentery

(D) diptheria

(E) disseminated intravascular coagulation

8. In people who have sickle cell anemia, osteomyelitis usually is associated with which of the following organisms?

(A) *Micrococcus*

(B) *Escherichia*

(C) *Pseudomonas*

(D) *Salmonella*

(E) *Streptococcus*

9. The sensitivity of LA is

(A) 0 percent

(B) 30 percent

(C) 85 percent

(D) 95 percent

(E) 100 percent

10. Choose the antibiotic therapy of choice for Legionellosis

(A) Penicillin

(B) Ampicillin

(C) Erythromycin

(D) Vancomycin

(E) Ceftriaxone

11. Which antibiotic inhibits dihydrofolate reductase

(A) Penicillin

(B) Amdinocillin

(C) Amphotericin

(D) Chloramphenicol

(E) Trimethroprim

12. *Escherichia coli* has two major porins located in the outer membrane. The function of porins is

(A) stabilization of the mesosome

(B) metabolism of phosphorylated intermediates

(C) transfer of small molecules through the outer membrane

(D) serologic stabilization of the O antigen

(E) diffusion of safranin from the cell, thereby rendering the cell gram-negative

13. In the immunologic technique, (ELISA), antigen undergoes electrophoresis through polacylamide gel and is transferred to nitrocellulose, where it is reacted with antisera. This is best described as:

(A) Affinity chromatography

(B) Radial immunodiffusion

(C) Rocket immunoelectrophoresis

(D) Western or immunoblot

(E) Enzyme-linked immunosorbent

14. Which of the following is a newly identified species of *Chlamydia* that causes acute respiratory disease in adults and is not associated with avian sources?

(A) *C. pneumoniae*

(B) *C. trachomatis*

(C) *C. psittaci*

(D) *C. lymphovenereum*

(E) *C. hominis*

15. An inhibitor of ATP synthesis would be expected to retard most severely the penetration of the host cell by which of the following organisms?

(A) *Chlamydia psittaci*

(B) *Chlamydia trachomatis*

(C) *Ureaplasma urealyticum*

(D) *Rickettsia rickettsii*

(E) *Mycoplasma pneumoniae*

16. The naming of fungi is very confusing to the nonmycologist. For this reason, the clinician who may treat fungal infections should have a working knowledge of fungal taxonomy. Most of the fungi known to cause infection in humans have been recognized for many years by their asexual stage (anamorph). The sexual stage (teleomorph) of many of these familiar fungi has now been discovered. Which is the appropriate lettered teleomorph for Trichophyton mentagrophytes

(A) *Ajellomyces capsulata*

(B) *Ajellomyces dermatitidis*

(C) *Arthroderma van breuseghemii*

(D) *Filobasidiella neoformans*

(E) *Nannizzia incurvata*

17. A 6-year old girl presented to the clinic with scaly patches on the scalp. Primary smears and culture of the skin and hair were negative. A few weeks later, she returned and was found to have inflammatory lesions. The hair fluoresced under Wood's light and primary smears of the skin and hair contained septate hyphae. On speaking with the parents, it was discovered that there were several pets in the household. Which of the following is the most likely agent?

(A) *Microporum audouini*

(B) *Microsporum canis*

(C) *Trichophyton tonsurans*

(D) *Trichophyton rubrum*

(E) *Epidermophyton floccosum*

18. Which of the following techniques is employed most successfully for recovering pinworm eggs?

(A) Sugar fecal flotation

(B) Zinc-sulfate fecal flotation

(C) Tap-water fecal sedimentation

(D) Direct fecal centrifugal flotation

(E) Anal swabbing with cellophane tape

19. A young girl has had repeated infections with Candida albicans and respiratory viruses since the time she was 3 months old. As part of the clinical evaluation of her immune status, her responses to routine immunization procedures should be tested. In this evaluation, the use of which of the following vaccines is contraindicated?

(A) Diptheria toxoid

(B) Bordetella pertussis vaccine

(C) Tetanus toxoid

(D) BCG

(E) Inactivated polio

20. Complement-fixation (CF) testing is an important serologic tool. What is the expected result for the reaction mixture: anti-Mycoplasma antibody + complement + hemolysin-sensitized red blood cells (RBC) + anti-RBC antibody

(A) Complement is bound, red blood cells are lysed

(B) Complement is bound, red blood cells are not lysed

(C) Complement is not bound, red blood cells are lysed

(D) Complement is not bound, red blood cells are not lysed

(E) Complement is not bound, red blood cells are agglutinated

21. Uptake by a recipient cell of soluble DNA released from a donor cell is most likely to be associated with

(A) Conjugation

(B) Recombination

(C) Competence

(D) Transformation

(E) Transduction

22. The diagnosis of fungal infection may be clinical, serologic, microscopic, or cultural. Although the isolation and identification of a fungus from a suspect lesion establishes a precise diagnosis, it is time-consuming. Microscopy is more rapid but generally less sensitive. Visualization of fungi in a clinical specimen is best accomplished by treatment of the specimen with

(A) silver nitrate

(B) hydrochloric acid

(C) potassium hydroxide

(D) para-aminobenzonic acid

(E) calcofluor white

23. A nurse develops clinical symptoms consistent with hepatitis. She recalls sticking herself with a needle approximately 4 months ago after drawing blood from a patient. Serologic tests for HBsAg, antibodies to HBsAg, and hepatitis A virus (HAV) are all negative; however, she is positive for IgM core antibody. The nurse

(A) does not have hepatitis B

(B) has hepatitis A

(C) is in the late stages of hepatitis B infection

(D) is in the "window" (after the disappearance of HBsAg and before the appearance of anti-HBsAg)

(E) has hepatitis C

24. Which organism is the causative agent of Rocky Mountain spotted fever

(A) *Rochalimaea quintana*

(B) *Coxiella burnetti*

(C) *Rickettsia rickettsii*

(D) *Chlamydia trachomatis*

(E) None of the above

25. A butcher, who is fond of eating raw hamburger, develops chorioetinitis. A Sabin-Feldman dye test is positive. What is the most likely diagnosis

(A) Trichinosis

(B) Schistosomiasis

(C) Toxoplasmosis

(D) Viseral larva migrans

(E) Giardiasis

MICROBIOLOGY II PRACTICE TEST

ANSWER SHEET

CUT HERE

	ANS	CON
1.		
2.		
3.		
4.		
5.		
6.		
7.		
8.		
9.		
10.		
11.		
12.		
13.		

	ANS	CON
14.		
15.		
16.		
17.		
18.		
19.		
20.		
21.		
22.		
23.		
24.		
25.		

SEE PAGE **25** FOR INSTRUCTIONS
SEE PAGE **213** FOR ANSWERS

STUDY SUGGESTION

When taking a test, pacing should be done on average; some questions require more time, others less.

Consider the issue on page 74. The statement is False.

MICROBIOLOGY II

1. All the following statements about human rotaviruses are true EXCEPT that they

(A) produce an infection that is seasonally distributed in temperate climates, peaking in fall and winter

(B) produce cytopathic effects in many conventional tissue culture systems

(C) are nonlipid-containing RNA viruses possessing a double-shelled capsid

(D) can be sensitively and rapidly detected in stools by the enzyme-linked immunosorbent assay (ELISA) technique

(E) have been implicated as a major etiologic agent of infantile gastroenteritis

2. A 19-year-old woman reports to the college infirmary with the chief complaint of frequency of urination and a burning sensation. She has some mild lower back pain. A urine sample is sent to the laboratory, where it is plated on blood agar (BAP) and MacConkey's (MAC) agar. The following day, there are approximately 30,000 cfu/ml on the BAP, nothing on the MAC. Gram's stain of the colonies shows gram-positive cocci in clumps. What is the most likely cause of the patient's urinary tract infection?

(A) *Staphylococcus aureus*

(B) *Staphylococcus epidermidis*

(C) *Staphylococcus saprophyticus*

(D) Group B streptococcus

(E) Pneumococcus

3. A 4-year-old child presents in the emergency room with a rash and illness characteristic of chickenpox. One member of the medical team attending this patient is a pregnant nurse with no history of chickenpox. The decision is made to administer zoster immune globulin to the nurse, but the suggestion is made that a serum sample be drawn prior to this to determine her true immune status. The test necessary to determine immune status for varicella-zoster virus is

(A) complement fixation

(B) fluorescent antibody to membrane antigen (FAMA)

(C) direct fluorescent antibody

(D) indirect fluorescent antibody

(E) enzyme immunoassay

4. Infection with Epstein-Barr virus (EBV) results in the development of virus-specific antibodies. In the case of infectious mononucleosis, for EBNA-Ab, choose the description with which it is most likely to be associated.

(A) Appears 2 weeks to several months after onset and is present more often in atypical cases of infectious mononucleosis

(B) Appears 3 to 4 weeks after onset; titers correlate with severity of clinical illness

(C) Arises early in the course of the illness; detectable titers persist a lifetime

(D) Appears late in the course of the disease and persists a lifetime

(E) Arises early in the course of the illness, and then titers fall rapidly

5. At a church supper in Nova Scotia, the following meal was served: baked beans, ham, coleslaw, eclairs, and coffee. Of the 30 people who attended, 4 senior citizens became ill in 3 days; 1 eventually died. Two weeks subsequent to the church supper, a 19-year-old girl who attended the supper gave birth to a baby who rapidly became ill with meningitis and died in 5 days. Epidemiologic investigation revealed the following percentages of people who consumed the various food items: baked beans 30 percent, ham 80 percent, coleslaw 60 percent, eclairs 100 percent, and coffee 90 percent. All the following statements are true EXCEPT

(A) this is not a case of food poisoning because only 4 people became ill

(B) the death of the baby may be related to the food consumed at the church supper

(C) based on the epidemiologic investigation, no one food item can be implicated as the cause of the disease

(D) additional data on the microbiologic analysis of the food are required

(E) additional epidemiologic data should include the percentage of those who ate a particular food item who became ill

6. Choose the source from which the vaccine for eastern equine encephalitis is obtained.

(A) Calf or sheep lymph

(B) Duck embryo

(C) Chick embryo cell culture

(D) Chick embryo tissue culture

(E) Monkey kidney tissue culture

7. The class of antibiotics known as the quinolones are bactericidal. Their mode of action on growing bacteria is thought to be

(A) inhibition of DNA gyrase

(B) inactivation of penicillin-binding protein II

(C) inhibition of b-lactamase

(D) prevention of the cross-linking of glycine

(E) inhibition of reverse transcriptase

8. A patient complained to his dentist about a draining lesion in his mouth. A Gram's stain of the pus showed a few gram-positive cocci, leukocytes, and many branched gram-positive rods. The most likely cause of the disease is

(A) *Actinomyces israelii*

(B) *Actinomyces viscosus*

(C) *Corynebacterium diphtheriae*

(D) *Propionibacterium acnes*

(E) *Staphylococcus aureus*

9. An obstetrician sees a pregnant patient who has been exposed to the rubella virus in the 18th week of gestation. She has no history of rubella and on serological testing has no detectable antibody. The best course of action would be to

(A) vaccinate her immediately

(B) administer rubella immune serum

(C) suggest termination of pregnancy

(D) follow her antibody titer serologically

(E) assure her that no problem exists because she is past the first trimester of pregnancy

10. Thrombocytopenic patients who have aplastic anemia benefit from platelet transfusions during periods of severe platelet depression. Platelets may be rejected because of an ABO or HL-A incompatibility. Which of the following platelet-transfusion donors would be best for a patient whose blood type is A- and HL-A haplotypes 1,3; 7,12?

(A) O— 1,3; 7,12
(B) A+   3,5; 7,8
(C) O— 3,5; 7,8
(D) AB— 2,—; 5,13
(E) A+   1,3; 7,12

11. Choose the lettered growth curve (in an exponentially growing culture) with which chloramphenicol is most likely to be associated. (The arrow in the graph indicates the time at which the drugs were added.)

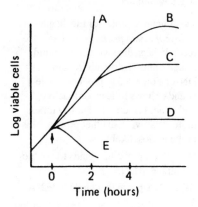

(A) A
(B) B
(C) C
(D) D
(E) E

12. A 21-year-old man was bitten by a tick in Oregon. Two years later, during the course of routine screening for an unknown ailment, a screening Lyme disease test was performed, which was negative. A western blot strip (IgG) showed the following pattern:

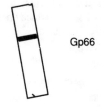

Gp66

Which of the following is the correct interpretation of the test?
(A) The patient has acute Lyme disease
(B) The patient has chronic Lyme disease
(C) The pattern may represent nonspecific reactivity
(D) The screening test should be repeated
(E) The patient should be tested for HIV on the basis of the western blot

13. Patients who have disseminated coccidioidomycosis may often demonstrate any of the following EXCEPT
(A) a positive coccidioidin skin test
(B) a negative coccidioidin skin test
(C) immunity to reinfection
(D) a high titer of complement-fixing (CF) antibodies
(E) a negative CF antibody test

14. Select the organism most likely to be the causative agent of the skin disease tinea corporis

(A) *Epidermophyton floccosum*

(B) *Malassezia furfur*

(C) *Microsporum canis*

(D) *Exophiala werneckii*

(E) *Trichosporon beigelii*

15. An ill patient denied being bitten by insects. However, he had spent some time in a milking barn and indicated that it was dusty. Of the following rickettsial diseases, which one has he most likely contracted?

(A) Scrub typhus

(B) Rickettsialpox

(C) Brill-Zinsser disease

(D) Q fever

(E) Rocky Mountain spotted fever

16. Chlamydiae have an unusual three-stage cycle of development. The correct sequence of these events is

(A) penetration of the host cell, synthesis of elementary body progeny, development of an initial body

(B) penetration of the host cell, development of an initial body, synthesis of elementary body progeny

(C) development of an initial body, synthesis of elementary body progeny, penetration of the host cell

(D) synthesis of elementary body progeny, development of an initial body, penetration of the host cell

(E) synthesis of elementary body progeny, penetration of the host cell, development of an initial body

17. A slide culture of a dematiacious mold revealed the image below. The most likely identity of this mold is

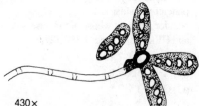

430×
Multicelled conidia (black) produced sympodially

(A) *Drechslera*

(B) *Cladosporium*

(C) *Alternaria*

(D) *Penicillium*

(E) *Acremonium*

18. A genetic probe for the diagnosis of *Mycoplasma pneumoniae* has recently been discovered. It is rapid (takes 2 hours), does not require that DNA be digested to produce single strands, shows little cross reactivity with other bacteria, and is 100 times more sensitive than other probes. This probe is most likely

(A) a DNA probe that binds to double-stranded DNA

(B) a DNA probe that binds to tRNA

(C) a DNA probe that is specific for the genus *Mycoplasma* and binds to cell-wall constituents

(D) an RNA probe that binds to ribosomal RNA

(E) an RNA probe that binds to mRNA

19. A woman who recently traveled through Central Africa now complains of severe chills and fever, abdominal tenderness, and darkening urine. Her febrile periods last for 28 hours and recur regularly. Which of the blood smears drawn below would be most likely to be associated with the symptoms described?

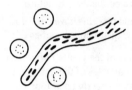

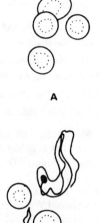

A   B

C

D

E

(A) A
(B) B
(C) C
(D) D
(E) E

20. Choose the preferred isolation medium for the bacteria, *Neisseria gonorrhoeae*.

(A) Sheep blood agar

(B) Löffler's medium

(C) Thayer-Martin agar

(D) Thiosulfate citrate bile salts sucrose medium

(E) Löwenstein-Jensen agar

21. All the following statements concerning immunoglobulin structure are true EXCEPT

(A) the amino acid sequence variation of the heavy chains is similar to that observed in light chains

(B) in man, there are approximately twice as many Ig molecules with κ and λ chains

(C) in the three-dimensional structure of Ig, there is little, if any, flexibility in the hinge region between the Fc and two Fab portions

(D) IgM is a pentameric structure

(E) myeloma proteins have been widely used for Ig structural studies

22. Members of the genus *Babesia* are sporozoan parasites of the red blood cell that have recently been found to cause human infections. Infection usually results in a febrile illness associated with hemolysis. Humans become infected from

(A) ticks

(B) mosquitoes

(C) fleas

(D) mites

(E) none of the above

23. A 3-year-old child presents at the physician's office with symptoms of coryza, conjuctivitis, low-grade fever, and Koplik's spots. The causative agent of this disease belongs to which group of viruses?

(A) Adenovirus

(B) Herpesvirus

(C) Picornavirus

(D) Orhtomyxovirus

(E) Paramyxovirus

24. A primary procedure for diagnosis of fecal parasites is a stained smear of feces. For some parasitic infections, however, other specimens may be more pro-ductive. What is the best method of identification for the parasite *Giardia lamblia* ?

(A) Sigmoidoscopy and aspiration of mucosal lesions

(B) Baermann technique

(C) Dilution followed by egg count

(D) Enzyme immunoassay (EIA)

(E) Examination of a cellophane tape swab

25. Most, but not all, cases of hepatitis are caused by hepatitis A virus (HAV), hepatitis B virus (HBV), or non-A, non-B hepatitis virus. While the laboratory diagnosis of HAV is usually accomplished by the detection of IgG and IgM antibodies to HAV, the diagnosis of HBV is more complex.. Match the correct HBV infection to the immunologic marker: IgG antibodies to core antigen, antibodies to E antigen, antibodies to surface antigen

(A) Acute infection (incubation period)

(B) Acute infection (acute phase)

(C) Post infection/exposure

(D) Immunization

(E) HBV carrier state

NEUROSCIENCE PRACTICE TEST

ANSWER SHEET

	ANS	CON			ANS	CON
1.				**14.**		
2.				**15.**		
3.				**16.**		
4.				**17.**		
5.				**18.**		
6.				**19.**		
7.				**20.**		
8.				**21.**		
9.				**22.**		
10.				**23.**		
11.				**24.**		
12.				**25.**		
13.						

SEE PAGE **25** FOR INSTRUCTIONS
SEE PAGE **214** FOR ANSWERS

CUT HERE

STUDY SUGGESTION

True or False:
When approaching a matching question, it is most productive and efficient to choose the same answer for two questions when you are experiencing pairwise confusion.

See page 94 for a discussion of this issue.

NEUROSCIENCE

Questions 1. - 4. Kuffler studied the electrophysiology of glial cells, using the optic nerve and its surrounding glial sheath. He found that the mean value of the resting potential of these cells, as recorded by intracellular microelectrodes, was –89.6 mV. The potassium concentration in the bathing solution was 3 mEq/L. Assume that RT/F = 61.

1. Assuming that the resting potential is equivalent to the potassium equilibrium potential, calculate the approximate intracellular potassium concentration (in mEq/L):

(A) 11
(B) 33
(C) 88
(D) 140
(E) 155

2. Stimulation of the optic nerve with a volley of impulses caused a slow and long-lasting depolarization of the associated glial cells. The mean value of the depolarization was 12.1 mV. If this depolarization was due solely to an increase in potassium ion concentration in the intracellular clefts, calculate the change in the concentration of potassium in the extracellular environment (in mEq/L).

(A) 1.79
(B) 36.30
(C) 137.00
(D) 140.50
(E) 5.35 x 10⁻⁶

3. What would be the concentration of potassium (mEq/L) in the bathing fluid in order to depolarize the membrane potential to zero?

(A) 11
(B) 33
(C) 88
(D) 140
(E) 155

4. A probable explanation for the depolarization of glial cells following stimulation of nerve fibers is that:

(A) it is a result of a delayed increase in potassium conductance
(B) it is a result of early sodium influx
(C) it is a result of a large efflux of sodium ions
(D) it is the product of temporal summation that results in a long-lasting depolarization
(E) it is a result of an influx of chloride ion

5. In Huntington's disease, there is a loss of:

(A) dopamine in the neostriatum
(B) substance P in the substantia nigra
(C) acetylcholine and gamma aminobutyric acid in intrastriatal and cortical neurons
(D) serotonin in the neostriatum
(E) most of the pallidal neurons

6. The Kluver-Bucy syndrome is typically associated with lesions of the:

(A) septal area
(B) amygdala
(C) cingulate gyrus
(D) medial hypothalamus
(E) lateral hypothalamus

DIRECTIONS: The questions below consist of lettered headings followed by a set of numbered items. For each numbered item select the **one** heading with which it is **most** closely associated. Each lettered heading may be used **once, more than once, or not at all.**

Questions 7. - 11.

(A) norepinephrine

(B) somatostatin

(C) cholecystokinin

(D) dopamine

(E) serotonin

(F) oxytocin

(G) gamma-aminobutyric acid (GABA)

(H) glycine

(I) enkephalins

(J) substance P

(K) glutamate

(L) acetylcholine

7. an inhibitory interneuron in the spinal cord

8. present in raphe neurons of the pons and caudal midbrain

9. present in the ventral tegmental and interpeduncular neurons of the midbrain

10. present in the locus ceruleus of the pons

11. present in the pars compacta of the substantia nigra

12. First-order sensory neurons that terminate in laminas I and II of the spinal cord convey mainly:

(A) tactile sensation

(B) pain and temperature sensation

(C) unconscious proprioception limited to inputs from muscle spindles

(D) unconscious proprioception limited to inputs from Golgi tendon organs

(E) inputs associated with pressure receptors

13. Which of the following statements concerning the zone of Lissauer is true:

(A) many fibers that convey unconscious proprioception enter this zone

(B) this zone is composed of coarse, heavily myelinated fibers

(C) fibers within the zone of Lissauer may ascend or descend several segments

(D) these fibers synapse with alpha motor neurons of extensor muscles

(E) cells in this zone typically project to thalamic nuclei

14. All the following play a role in the mediation or modulation of pain EXCEPT:

(A) neurons within the lateral hypothalamus

(B) substance P at primary afferent terminals

(C) opiate receptors in the spinal cord and brainstem

(D) neurons within the substantia gelatinosa

(E) neurons within the midbrain periaqueductal gray

15. Which of the following statements concerning the nucleus dorsalis of Clarke is correct:

(A) it is generally regarded as a nucleus associated with autonomic functions

(B) it contains second-order neurons for the transmission of unconscious proprioceptive information

(C) it contains second-order neurons for the transmission of information from pain receptors

(D) fibers originating from this nucleus cross in the spinal cord

(E) this nucleus is found principally at cervical levels of the cord

DIRECTIONS: The questions below consist of lettered headings followed by a set of numbered items. For each numbered item select the **one** heading with which it is **most** closely associated. Each lettered heading may be used **once, more than once, or not at all.**

Questions 16. - 19.

(A) special somatic afferent (SSA)

(B) special visceral afferent (SVA)

(C) general somatic afferent (GSA)

(D) general visceral afferent (GVA)

(E) general visceral efferent (GVE)

(F) special visceral efferent (SVE)

(G) general somatic efferent (GSE)

16. spiral ganglion

17. Scarpa's (vestibular) ganglion

18. superior salivatory nucleus

19. motor nucleus of cranial nerve V

20. All of the following statements concerning the inferior olivary complex are correct EXCEPT:

(A) It receives descending inputs from the red nucleus.

(B) Descending inputs come from the cerebral cortex.

(C) It receives direct inputs from ascending spinal fibers.

(D) Fibers arising from the inferior olivary nucleus project to the contralateral cerebellum via the inferior cerebellar peduncle.

(E) Inputs into cerebellum from the inferior olivary nucleus comprise part of the mossy fiber system.

21. Neurons capable of responding to the direction or orientation of a given stimulus moved along a receptive field are located in:

(A) spinal cord

(B) medulla

(C) pons

(D) thalamus

(E) cerebral cortex

22. In the olfactory glomerulus, primary afferent fibers terminate principally upon:

(A) granule cell dendrites forming axo-dendritic synapses

(B) granule cell axon terminals forming axo-axonic synapses

(C) mitral cell dendrites forming axo-dendritic synapses

(D) mitral cell axon terminals forming axo-axonic synapses

(E) axon terminals of fibers arising from the olfactory tubercle, forming axo-axonic synapses

23. Tardive dyskinesia is most likely the result of:

(A) a change in serotonin receptors causing a hypersensitivity to serotonin

(B) a change in acetylcholine receptors causing a hypersensitivity to acetylcholine

(C) a change in enkephalin receptors causing a hypersensitivity to enkephalin

(D) a change in dopamine receptors causing a hypersensitivity to dopamine

(E) a change in gamma amino butyric acid (GABA) receptors causing a hypersensitivity to GABA

24. The amygdala receives significant inputs from all of the following structures EXCEPT:

(A) prefrontal cortex

(B) cingulate gyrus

(C) hypothalamus

(D) locus ceruleus

(E) olfactory bulb

25. All of the following statements concerning the dorsal columns are true EXCEPT:

(A) they contain first-order neurons which synapse in contralateral dorsal column nuclei

(B) they contain first-order neurons mediating conscious proprioception from the limbs

(C) sensation from the lower limb is contained in the fasciculus gracilis while sensation from the upper limb is contained in the fasciculus cuneatus

(D) a lesion of the fasciculus gracilis may result in ataxia

(E) they contain fibers mediating either tactile or kinesthetic sensations, but not both

PATHOLOGY I PRACTICE TEST

ANSWER SHEET

	ANS	CON			ANS	CON
1.				14.		
2.				15.		
3.				16.		
4.				17.		
5.				18.		
6.				19.		
7.				20.		
8.				21.		
9.				22.		
10.				23.		
11.				24.		
12.				25.		
13.						

SEE PAGE 25 FOR INSTRUCTIONS
SEE PAGE 214 FOR ANSWERS

CUT HERE

STUDY SUGGESTION

When approaching a matching question, it is most productive and efficient to choose the same answer for two questions when you are experiencing pairwise confusion. You will be sure to get at least one of the two right.

Review Chapter 8 for further discussion of these recommendations.

Consider the issue on page 88. The statement is True.

PATHOLOGY I

1. Which group of factors is most important in the cellular pathogenesis of acute ischemia?

(A) Mitochondrial hyperplasia, lysozyme release, membrane injury

(B) Reduced ATP, increased calcium influx, membrane injury

(C) Lipid deposition, reduced protein synthesis, nuclear damage

(D) Ribosome detachment, glycolysis, nuclear damage

(E) Mitochondrial condensation, glycolysis, sodium cell loss

2. A young woman succumbed after an 8-month course of severe dyspnea, fatigue, and cyanosis that followed an uneventful delivery of a healthy infant. At necropsy, small atheromas were present in the large and small branches of the pulmonary arteries. Which of the following findings can be predicted in the histologic slides of the lungs?

(A) Diffuse hemorrhage and infarctions

(B) Diffuse alvelor hyaline membranes

(C) Severe atelectasis and edema

(D) Marked medial hypertrophy of pulmonary arterioles

(E) Multiple pulmonary emboli

3. In which disease is hyperplastic arteriolar nephrosclerosis most characteristic.

(A) Malignant hypertension

(B) Systemic lupus erthematosus

(C) Chronic thyroiditis

(D) Addison's disease

(E) Diabetic anephropathy

4. The cluster of cells in the photomicrograph below appeared in cytologic specimen of sputum from a 57-year-old man with chest pain, memoptysis, and a nonproductive cough of many years' duration. Which of the following is the most likely diagnosis?

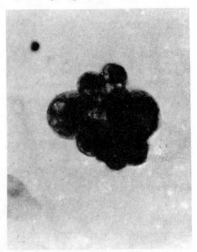

(A) Squamous cell metaplasia of ciliated, bronchial epithelium

(B) Oat cell (small-cell undifferentiated) carcinoma

(C) Adenocarcinoma

(D) Cytomegalic inclusion virus pneumonia

(E) Normal bronchial epithelium

5. Which of the following conditions is most likely to predispose to thrombosis and embolism?

(A) Atrial fibrillation

(B) Pulmonary stenosis

(C) Ventricular septal defect

(D) Aortic stenosis

(E) Atrial septal defect

6. A young child has recurrent bacterial infections, eczema, thrombocytopenia, lymphadenopathy, and the absence of delayed-type hypersensitivity. The most likely diagnosis is

(A) Pelger-Huet anomaly

(B) Wiskott-Aldrich syndrome

(C) Chediak-Higashi syndrome

(D) chronic granulomatous disease of childhood

(E) nodular-sclerosing Hodgkin's disease

7. An elderly man treated for congestive heart failure for years with digitalis and furosemide dies of pulmonary edema. A postmortem examination of the heart would most likely show

(A) severe left ventricular hypertrophy

(B) right and left ventricular hypertrophy

(C) right ventricular infarction

(D) aortic and mitral valve stenosis

(E) a dilated, globular heart with thin walls

---

8. Acute lymphoblastic leukemia was diagnosed in a 10-year-old child, When this child later developed a patchy pulmonary infiltrate and respiratory insufficiency, a lung biopsy was performed. The material obtained by biopsy was then stained with Gomori's methenamine-silver stain and is shown in the photomicrograph below. In consideration of the patient's signs and microscopic evaluations, the prognosis is now complicated by

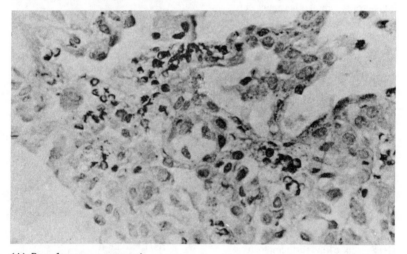

(A) *Pseudomonas* pneumonia

(B) *Aspergillus* pneumonia

(C) *Pneumocytis carinii* pneumonia

(D) pneumococcal pneumonia

(E) influenza pneumonia

9. What is the most likely cause of the malabsorption syndrome with a clinical and pathological pattern of recent viral infection, persistent diarrhea, and normal bowel mucosa

(A) Abetalipoproteinemia

(B) Primary intestinal lymphoma

(C) Whipple's disease

(D) Disaccharidase deficiency

(E) Systemic mastocytosis

10. What is the most characteristic finding of the respiratory disorder, Wegener's granulomatosis

(A) Myasthenic syndrome

(B) Fungal infection

(C) Hemorrhagic interstitial pneumonitis

(D) Nasal mucosal ulcerations

(E) Asthmatic bronchitis

11. A 25-year-old teacher was well until she went to a bazaar and ate barbecued turkey. The next day she had bloody diarrhea, crampy pain, and tenesmus. A gastroenterologist who did not take a history took a colon biopsy specimen that showed mucosal edema, congestion, and numerous lymphoid cells in the lamina propria. Which of the following differential diagnoses would apply?

(A) Staphylococcal gastroenteritis vs. Crohn's disease

(B) Viral gastroenteritis vs. acute diverticulitis

(C) Colonic endometriosis vs. amebic dysentery

(D) Early ulcerative colitis vs. Salmonella colitis

(E) Bleeding hemorrhoids vs. Meckel's diverticulitis

12. A 23-year-old woman with an abnormal Pap smear undergoes a cervical biopsy. The results are read as "CIN-2." What is the meaning of this report.

(A) Cervical carcinoma, grade II

(B) Cervical carcinoma, stage II

(C) Cervical inflammation; repeat in 2 months

(D) Carcinoma in situ

(E) Moderate dysplasia

13. A 10-year-old boy has a bout of ordinary upper respiratory infection followed within 36 hours by an episode of hematuria. There are no joint symptoms, gastrointestinal symptoms, petechiae, or rashes. To confirm Berger's disease, which of the following is indicated?

(A) Examination of urinary sediment

(B) Renal scan

(C) Renal biopsy immunofluorescence

(D) Creatinine clearance

(E) Intravenous pyelogram

14. With which sign is familial Alzheimer's disease most likely to be associated.

(A) Accumulation of GM2 ganglioside

(B) Genetic defect on chromosome 21

(C) Primary CNS demyelination

(D) Abnormal or defective myelin metabolism

(E) Genetic defect on chromosome 4

15. Which immunoglobulin with which it is most likely to be associated with anaphylaxis

(A) IgA

(B) IgD

(C) IgE

(D) IgM

(E) IgG

16. Tuberculous spondylitis (Pott's disease) is characterized by all of the following EXCEPT

(A) involvement of thoracic and lumbar vertebrae

(B) hematogenous spread

(C) proliferative synovitis with pannus

(D) destruction of intervertebral disks

(E) formation of psoas abscess

17. What is the creatinine clearance of a person who passes 361 mg of creatinine in a 24-hour urine sample of 77 ml and whose plasma creatinine is 2.0 mg/100 ml?

(A) 12.5 ml/min

(B) 25.0 ml/min

(C) 50.0 ml/min

(D) 75.0 ml/min

(E) 100.0 ml/min

18. All the following statements apply to ependymomas EXCEPT that

(A) they are the most common type of intraspinal glioma

(B) they are the most common primary brain tumor in children

(C) patients may present with headache and papilledema

(D) they may require differentiation from choroid plexus papilloma

(E) histologic sections display rosettes

19. With which sign is postencephalitic Parkinsonism most likely to be associated

(A) Neurofibrillary tangles

(B) Cowdry A intranuclear inclusions

(C) Optic nerve demyelination

(D) Hepatolenticular degeneration

(E) Verocay bodies

20. Osteogenesis imperfecta type I is characterized by

(A) a hereditary defect in osteoclast function

(B) defective synthesis of type II collagen

(C) defective synthesis of osteoid matrix

(D) early death

(E) bone marrow aplasia

21. Which of the following cell populations of the central nervous system is the most rapidly affected by ischemia?

(A) Axis cylinders

(B) Neuronal nerve cell bodies

(C) Astrocytes

(D) Microglia

(E) Oligodendroglia

22. In tissues affected by the predominant form of Niemann-Pick disease, which of the following is found at abnormally high levels?

(A) Sphingomyelin

(B) Sphingomyelinase

(C) Kerasin

(D) Acetyl coenzyme A

(E) Ganglioside

23. A 42-year-old man complains of recently having to change his shoe size from 9 to 10-1/2, and he also says that his hands and jaw are now larger. The disorder is most likely mediated through

(A) prolactin

(B) ACTH

(C) somatomedin

(D) antidiuretic hormone

(E) thyrotropin

24. A 56-year-old woman has for 1 year's duration indurated plaques and nodules about the lower back and proximal thighs; the skin biopsy is seen below. What nuclear features are characteristic for this disorder?

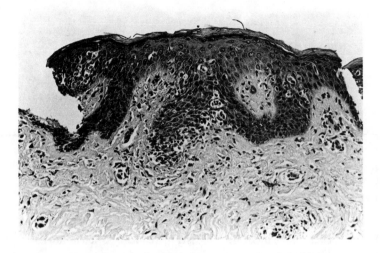

(A) Markedly thickened nuclear membranes

(B) Unusually large nucleoli

(C) Folded, cerebriform nuclei

(D) Numerous mitotic figures

(E) Nuclear pyknosis

25. A 20-year-old man presents in the emergency room with a lymphoma involving the mediastinum that is producing respiratory distress. The lymphocytes are most likely to have cell surface markers characteristic of which of the following?

(A) B cells

(B) T cells

(C) Macrophages

(D) Dendritic reticulum cells

(E) Langerhans cells

STUDY SUGGESTION

Try answering this question:

A behavior pattern that increases in frequency when followed by a reward is an example of

- A. Classical conditioning
- B. Shaping
- C. Respondent conditioning
- D. Operant conditioning
- E. Generalization

See page 102 for a discussion of this question.

PATHOLOGY II PRACTICE TEST

ANSWER SHEET

	ANS	CON
1.		
2.		
3.		
4.		
5.		
6.		
7.		
8.		
9.		
10.		
11.		
12.		
13.		

	ANS	CON
14.		
15.		
16.		
17.		
18.		
19.		
20.		
21.		
22.		
23.		
24.		
25.		

SEE PAGE **25** FOR INSTRUCTIONS
SEE PAGE **214** FOR ANSWERS

CUT HERE

STUDY SUGGESTION

As you review, always test whether or not you can recall the information that is presented in your source. Use practice questions to evaluate your knowledge on a regular basis.

**ANSWER TO THE QUESTION
ON PAGE 100**

Can you reword this question so that the correct answer is "A. Classical conditioning?" What is shaping; generalization? Can you think of an example for each? If you know the answer to the main question but not to these other questions, you need to learn more. Understand all the alternatives if you want to benefit maximally from using practice questions as you review.

(See **Behavioral Science: PreTest®,** 5th ed., #151, p. 68.)

PATHOLOGY II

1. In tissues affected by the predominant form of Niemann-Pick disease, which of the following is found at abnormally high levels?

(A) Sphingomyelin

(B) Sphingomyelinase

(C) Kerasin

(D) Acetyl coenzyme A

(E) Ganglioside

2. True statements concerning diagnostic specificity include all the following EXCEPT

(A) Scl-70 antibody is specific for diffuse systemic sclerosis

(B) antibodies to nucleolar RNA are specific for diffuse systemicsclerosis

(C) antibodies to double-stranded DNA are specific for systemic lupus erythematosus (SLE)

(D) antibodies to antinuclear antibody (ANA) are specific for SLE

(E) anti-Sm antibodies are specific for SLE

3. The "stat" laboratory sends the following electrolyte results to the ward concerning a new admission: Na^+, 142 mEq/L; K^+, 7.2 mEq/L; Cl^-, 101 mEq/L; and CO_2, 32 mEq/L. On the basis of these results, the physician should

(A) treat with sodium exchange resin

(B) institute peritoneal dialysis immediately

(C) inquire about a hemolyzed blood sample

(D) infuse insulin intravenously

(E) make a diagnosis of hyperkalemia

4. The photomicrograph below is of peripheral blood from a patient with splenomegaly, anemia, and pancytopenia. If hairy cell leukemia is suspected, which of the following would be useful in establishing the diagnosis?

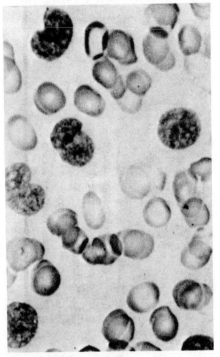

(A) Myeloperoxidase stain

(B) Sudan black B

(C) Acid phosphatase stain

(D) Leukocyte alkaline phosphatase

(E) Nonspecific esterase

5. Transferrin shows all the following characteristics EXCEPT

(A) normally about 33 percent saturation with iron

(B) increased saturation in hemochromatosis

(C) increased saturation in severe liver disease

(D) decreased saturation in marrow hypoplasia

(E) decreased saturation in iron deficiency anemia

6. A 48-year-old woman with a 26 pack-year history of cigarette smoking was noted to have abnormal cells (malignancy is suspected) in sputum cytology. The chest x-ray is presented. What is the most likely diagnosis?

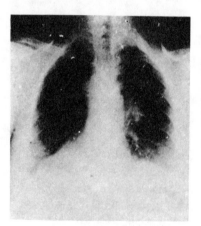

(A) Sarcoidosis

(B) Adenocarcinoma

(C) Breast carcinoma

(D) Small-cell carcinoma

(E) Squamous cell carcinoma

7. A 56-year-old woman died in a hospital where she was being evaluated for shortness of breath, ankle edema, and mild hepatomegaly. Because of the gross appearance of the liver at necropsy in the photograph below, one would also expect to find

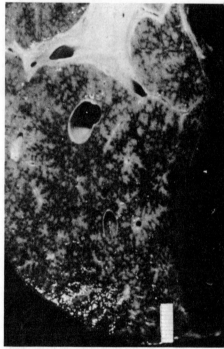

(A) a pulmonary saddle embolus

(B) right heart dilatation

(C) portal vein thrombosis

(D) biliary cirrhosis

(E) splenic amyloidosis

8. Which type of leukemia can be described by auer rods being frequently present in the leukemic cells?

(A) Acute lymphoblastic leukemia

(B) Acute myeloblastic leukemia (Ml)

(C) Acute promyelocytic leukemia (M3)

(D) Chronic lymphocytic leukemia

(E) Hairy cell leukemia

9. Choose the infectious agent that is most likely to be associated with the cardiac condition primary myocarditis.

(A) *Coxsackievirus*

(B) *Mycobacterium tuberculosis*

(C) *Streptococcus*

(D) *Treponema*

(E) *Escherichia coli*

10. Horner's syndrome is associated with

(A) lymphangitis carcinomatosa

(B) bronchial carcinoid

(C) exophthalmos

(D) tumor of the superior sulcus

(E) thoracocervical venous dilation

11. Two subtotal colectomy specimens are sent to the laboratory with both showing a hemorrhagic cobblestone appearance of the mucosa. One, however, shows longitudinal grooving of the surface, which suggests

(A) ischemic bowel disease

(B) multiple polyposis syndrome

(C) ulcerative colitis

(D) Crohn's disease

(E) none of the above

12. Choose the most common site of origin for the tumor, bronchial carcinoid

(A) Nasal cavity

(B) Neuroendocrine cells of bronchi

(C) Submucosal bronchial glands

(D) Terminal bronchioles

(E) Bronchial blood vessels

13. All the following statements regarding carcinoma of the esophagus are true EXCEPT

(A) most carcinomas arising in the body of the esophagus are squamous

(B) squamous carcinomas begin as lesions in situ

(C) patients with Barrett's esophagus have approximately a 10 percent risk of carcinoma

(D) the most common morphologic form is a polypoid fungating mass

(E) distant metastases are frequently present at the time of diagnosis

14. A middle-aged patient is undergoing surgical exploration for a tumor in the pancreatic fundus. No clinical history is given to the pathologist, who notes that the tumor has an "endocrine" appearance in frozen section. An appropriate step in the subsequent evaluation would be to consider

(A) immunoperoxidase

(B) brain scans

(C) computerized tomography

(D) celiac angiography

(E) immunofluorescence testing

15. All the following statements are true of urinary calculi EXCEPT that

(A) they are more common in males than in females

(B) they are bilateral in 40 percent of cases

(C) they are radiopaque in about 90 percent of cases

(D) they may be associated with *Pseudomonas* infections

(E) the incidence is increased in leukemia

16. An adult medical laboratory technician recovering from hepatitis B develops hematuria, proteinuria, and red cell casts in the urine. Which of the following would best describe the changes occurring within the kidney in this patient?

(A) Plasma cell interstitial nephritis

(B) IgG linear fluorescence along the glomerular basement membrane

(C) Granular deposits of antibodies in the glomerular basement membrane

(D) Diffuse glomerular basement membrane thickening by subepithelial immune deposits

(E) Nodular hyaline glomerulosclerosis

17. A 9-year-old boy who had been suffering from a gait disturbance for several weeks was found to have a posterior fossa mass on CT scan. The most likely cause for these findings is

(A) a berry aneurysm

(B) astrocytoma

(C) medulloblastoma

(D) oligodendroglioma

(E) pseudotumor cerebri

18. The photomicrograph below is of a section from a testis removed from the inguinal region of a man aged 25. Which of the following statements is true regarding the condition illustrated?

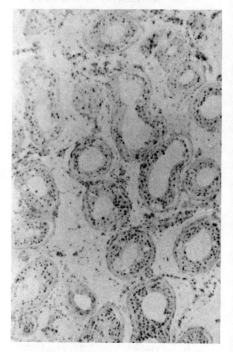

(A) It occurs in 5 percent of the adult male population

(B) Teratoma is the most common malignancy to arise

(C) Risk of associated malignancy is reduced by orchiopexy

(D) There is increased risk of malignancy in the contralateral testis

(E) Both Leydig and Sertoli cells are reduced in number

19. The most common etiologic factor in Cushing's syndrome is

(A) adrenal adenoma

(B) bilateral adrenal hyperplasia

(C) adrenal carcinoma

(D) ectopic adrenal tissue

(E) hypercorticism secondary to nonendocrine malignant tumors

20. All the following diseases may be associated with the grossly deformed joint depicted in the photograph below EXCEPT

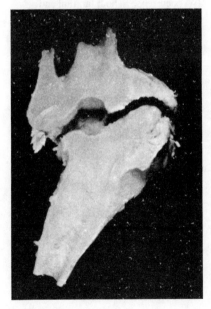

(A) leprosy

(B) psoriasis

(C) syringomyelia

(D) pernicious anemia

(E) diabetes mellitus

21. The specimen shown in the photomicrograph below is from a mass removed from the thigh of a 58-year-old man. Using the current nomenclature, this lesion is compatible with

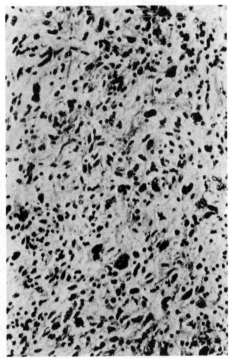

(A) nodular fasciitis

(B) rhabdomyosarcoma

(C) myositis ossificans

(D) osteogenic sarcoma

(E) malignant fibrous histiocytoma

22. Select the disorder below that has the most clinicopathologic features in common with postvaccinal encephalomyelitis.

(A) Metachromatic leukodystrophy

(B) Multifocal leukoencephalopathy

(C) Guillain-Barre syndrome

(D) Hypoxic encephalopathy

(E) Hypertensive encephalopathy

23. Which of the following statements most accurately describes inflammatory breast cancer?

(A) Inflammation improves the prognosis

(B) Inflammation is increased in Paget's disease

(C) Acute inflammatory cells are present

(D) Chronic inflammatory cells are present

(E) Lymphatic permeation is present

24. Which of the following cells can be described as having Ia and T6 surface membrane antigens?

(A) Merkel's cell

(B) Langerhans' cell

(C) Basal melanocyte

(D) Stratum basale cell

(E) Keratinocyte

25. Retinoblastoma, the most common intraocular tumor of children, is associated with all the following EXCEPT

(A) occurrence in both familial and sporadic patterns

(B) unilateral and unifocal sporadic tumors

(C) inactivation of cancer suppressor genes

(D) poor prognosis even with treatment

(E) frequent histologic occurrence of rosettes

PHARMACOLOGY I PRACTICE TEST

ANSWER SHEET

	ANS	CON			ANS	CON
1.				14.		
2.				15.		
3.				16.		
4.				17.		
5.				18.		
6.				19.		
7.				20.		
8.				21.		
9.				22.		
10.				23.		
11.				24.		
12.				25.		
13.						

CUT HERE

SEE PAGE 25 FOR INSTRUCTIONS
SEE PAGE 215 FOR ANSWERS

STUDY SUGGESTION

Frequent self-testing identifies topics most prone to forgetting. Self-testing also helps maintain knowledge by acting to refresh your memory.

PHARMACOLOGY I

1. If a drug is repeatedly administered at dosing intervals equal to its elimination half-life, the number of doses required for the plasma concentration of the drug to reach the steady state is

(A) 2 to 3
(B) 4 to 5
(C) 6 to 7
(D) 8 to 9
(E) 10 or more

2. Vertigo, inability to perceive termination of movement, and difficulty in sitting or standing without visual clues are some of the toxic reactions that are likely to occur in about 75 percent of patients who

(A) are allergic to penicillin
(B) receive tetracycline therapy
(C) receive amphotericin B therapy
(D) receive streptomycin therapy
(E) receive isoniazid therapy for tuberculosis

3. All the following statements are true about triazolam EXCEPT

(A) it binds to benzodiazepine receptor, enhancing GABA-mediated chloride influx
(B) it is useful in the treatment of insomnia
(C) it enhances the activity of the drug-metabolizing microsomal system
(D) combined with ethanol, it may produce significant respiratory depression
(E) adverse effects may include drowsiness, dizziness, lethargy, and ataxia

4. Convulsions caused by drug poisoning are most commonly associated with

(A) phenobarbital
(B) diazepam
(C) strychnine
(D) chlorpromazine
(E) phenytoin

5. All the following statements regarding the chemotherapy of cancer are true EXCEPT

(A) 50 percent of all newly diagnosed cancer patients will be cured
(B) chemotherapy is the only treatment that can effectively treat systemic disease
(C) chemotherapy only kills cancer cells and not normal dividing cells
(D) chemotherapy possesses numerous side effects, such as nausea, vomiting, and suppression of bone marrow
(E) new agents are cell-cycle specific

6. For the antibiotic Streptomycin, select the appropriate mode of action.

(A) Binds to the 30s ribosome subunit
(B) Inhibits binding of aminoacyl RNA to 50s ribosome subunit
(C) Inhibits production of cell wall
(D) Reversibly binds to 50s ribosome subunit
(E) Inhibits synthesis of steroids

7. In a nursing mother on sulfonamides, select the potential toxicity to the neonate.

(A) Pyridoxine deficiency
(B) Kernicterus
(C) Suppression of thyroid function
(D) Staining of developing teeth
(E) Sedation

8. What ist the most suitable description for benzathine penicillin G?

(A) Parenteral penicillin that is resistant to B-lactamase

(B) Referred to as an extended-spectrum penicillin

(C) Related to ampicillin but with better oral absorption

(D) Administered intramuscularly and yields prolonged drug levels

(E) Given parenterally and may cause elevation of serum sodium

9. Which of the following is an antidepressant agent that selectively inhibits serotonin (5-HT) uptake with minimal effect on norepinephrine uptake?

(A) Protriptyline

(B) Maprotiline

(C) Fluoxetine

(D) Desipramine

(E) Amoxapine

10. Which of the following drugs does not cross the placenta and has no significant concentration in milk in the lactating female?

(A) Heparin

(B) Dicumarol

(C) Warfarin

(D) Phenindione

(E) Acenocoumarol

11. Hyperkalemia is a contraindication to the use of which of the following drugs?

(A) Acetazolamide (Diamox)

(B) Chlorothiazide (Diuril)

(C) Ethacrynic acid (Edecrin)

(D) Chlorthalidone (Hygroton)

(E) Spironolactone (Aldactone)

12. Methyldopa (Aldomet) is an antihypertensive agent that acts by

(A) blocking β-adrenergic receptors

(B) preventing conversion of angiotensinogen to angiotensin

(C) stimulating α-adrenergic receptors in the central nervous system

(D) directly dilating arteriolar smooth muscle

(E) producing catecholamine depletion at postganglionic sympathetic nerves

13. Many drugs are associated with an ability to induce physical dependence as well as a craving for and tolerance to their psychological effects. Choose the effect that Meperidine usually produces

(A) Psychic dependence

(B) Tachyphylaxis

(C) Physical dependence only

(D) Tolerance and physical dependence

(E) None of the above

14. If both quinidine and digoxin are administered concurrently, which of the following effects does quinidine have on digoxin?

(A) The absorption of digoxin from the GI tract is decreased

(B) The metabolism of digoxin is prevented

(C) The concentration of digoxin in the plasma is increased

(D) The effect of digoxin on the AV node is antagonized

(E) The ability of digoxin to inhibit the Na^+, K^+ -stimulated ATPase is reduced

15. The mechanism of action of the long-lasting organic phosphate anticholinesterases is

(A) splitting of polypeptide bonds in cholinesterases

(B) phosphorylation of the anionic site of cholinesterases

(C) phosphorylation of the esteratic site of cholinesterases

(D) acetylation of the anionic site of cholinesterases

(E) acetylation of the esteratic site of cholinesterases

16. The effect of tranylcypromine can be attributed to

(A) a direct nicotine-like stimulation

(B) inhibition of serotonin uptake

(C) a xanthine-like stimulation

(D) the inhibition of monoamine oxidase

(E) blockade of dopamine receptors

17. The preferred thyroid prepar-ation for maintenance replacement therapy is which of the following drugs?

(A) Desiccated thyroid

(B) Liothyronine (Cytomel)

(C) Protirelin (Thypinone)

(D) Levothyroxine (Levothroid)

(E) Liotrix (Euthroid)

18. Norfloxacin acid, a quinolone derivative, is

(A) effective in the treatment of urinary tract infections

(B) effective in preventing cell-wall synthesis

(C) ineffective against *Pseudomonas aeruginosa*

(D) only administered parenterally

(E) a nonhalogenated derivative

19. A reduction in insulin release from the pancreas may be caused by which of the following diuretics?

(A) Triamterene (Dyrenium)

(B) Chlorothiazide (Diuril)

(C) Spironolactone (Aldactone)

(D) Acetazolamide (Diamox)

(E) Amiloride (Midamor)

20. The release of antidiuretic hormone (ADH) is suppressed by which of the following drugs to promote a diuresis?

(A) Guanethidine (Ismelin)

(B) Acetazolamide (Diamox)

(C) Chlorothiazide (Diuril)

(D) Ethanol

(E) Indomethacin (Indocin)

21. Metyrapone is useful in testing the endocrine functioning of the

(A) α cells of pancreatic islets

(B) β cells of pancreatic islets

(C) neurohypophysis

(D) pituitary-adrenal axis

(E) Leydig cells of testes

22. Rantidine (Zantac) is effective in treating duodenal ulcer because it

(A) strengthens the protective coating on the intestinal wall

(B) reduces parasympathetic-induced gastrointestinal secretions by competing at muscarinic receptors

(C) is an agonist at H_1 receptors and therefore reduces pepsin secretion

(D) blocks histamine stimulation of gastric acid secretion by H_2 receptors

(E) increases bicarbonate ion secretion, neutralizing the pH

23. Abuse of anabolic steroids by athletes can result in all the following EXCEPT

(A) retention of fluid

(B) feminization in males

(C) decreased spermatogenesis

(D) depression

(E) anorexia

24. Drugs may be released slowly from various drug reservoirs over long periods of time. The body reservoir that holds the largest amount of the barbiturate thiopental (Pentothal) is

(A) fat

(B) lung

(C) liver

(D) muscle

(E) serum albumin

25. The drug most effective against malarial parasites in the liver but not against parasites within erythrocytes is

(A) primaquine

(B) pyrimethamine

(C) quinacrine

(D) chloroquine

(E) chloroguanide

PHARMACOLOGY II PRACTICE TEST
ANSWER SHEET

	ANS	CON			ANS	CON
1.				**14.**		
2.				**15.**		
3.				**16.**		
4.				**17.**		
5.				**18.**		
6.				**19.**		
7.				**20.**		
8.				**21.**		
9.				**22.**		
10.				**23.**		
11.				**24.**		
12.				**25.**		
13.						

SEE PAGE **25** FOR INSTRUCTIONS
SEE PAGE **215** FOR ANSWERS

CUT HERE

STUDY SUGGESTION

Study as if for an essay examination as opposed to a multiple-choice examination. This forces you to organize and summarize your knowledge into coherent bodies of information as opposed to learning lists of facts. Research shows that preparing for an essay examination leads to significantly better performance on multiple-choice examinations than does preparing for a multiple-choice examination itself.

PHARMACOLOGY II

1. Drugs may be released slowly from various drug reservoirs over long periods of time. The body reservoir that holds the largest amount of the barbiturate thiopental (Pentothal) is

(A) fat

(B) lung

(C) liver

(D) muscle

(E) serum albumin

2. Select the characteristic that is most likely to be associated with streptozotocin.

(A) Used in treatment of Hodgkin's lymphoma

(B) Orally administered alkylating agent

(C) Retained specifically in beta cells of the islets of Langerhans

(D) Useful as a single agent against malignant melanoma

(E) An antitumor antibiotic that results in a high incidence of bone marrow suppression

3. Isoniazid, one of the most active drugs for the treatment of tuberculosis,

(A) cannot be used with rifampin or ethambutol

(B) works primarily by preventing protein synthesis

(C) possesses toxicities that can be prevented by pyridoxine

(D) is removed from the body un-changed

(E) is rarely met with resistance to its action

4. Receptors that have been activated by neurotransmitters or hormones initiate the formation or accumulation of intracellular second messengers that may include all the following EXCEPT

(A) cyclic AMP

(B) ACTH (corticotropin)

(C) diacylglycerol

(D) ionic calcium

(E) inositol-1,4,5-triphosphate

5. The drug most effective against malarial parasites in the liver but not effective against parasites within erythrocytes is

(A) primaquine

(B) pyrimethamine

(D) quinacrine

(D) chloroquine

(E) chloroguanide

6. The mechanism of action by which niclosamide is effective against adult intestinal cestodes is

(A) interference with cell-wall synthesis

(B) interference with cell division

(C) inhibition of mitochondrial oxidative phosphorylation

(D) interference with protein synthesis

(E) depletion of membrane lipoproteins

7. Which of the following local anesthetics is *only* useful for topical (surface) administration?

(A) Procaine

(B) Bupivacaine

(C) Etidocaine

(D) Benzocaine

(E) Lidocaine

8. Select the pair of substances that illustrates therapeutic interaction with a *reduction* in drug effectiveness.

(A) Tetracycline and milk

(B) Amobarbital (Amytal) and secobarbital (Seconal)

(C) Isoproterenol (Isuprel) and propranolol (Inderal)

(D) Soap and benzalkonium chloride (Ionil)

(E) Sulfamethoxazole and trimethoprim

9. A 24-year-old man is brought to the emergency room by a group of friends who said that he had suddenly become restless, confused, and uncoordinated after taking some pills. Physical examination reveals increased body temperature, tachycardia, cutaneous flush, and widely dilated pupils unresponsive to light. The patient complains of dryness of the mouth. He probably ingested which of the following drugs?

(A) Codeine

(B) Aspirin

(C) Secobarbital

(D) Atropine

(E) Chlordiazepoxide

10. Many drugs, when given to a pregnant woman, produce significant adverse effects on the fetus. For the drug diethylstilbestrol, match the most appropriate adverse effect.

(A) Vaginal adenocarcinoma

(B) Congenital goiter, hypothyroidism

(C) Masculinization of female fetus

(D) Gray baby syndrome

(E) Prolonged neonatal hypoglycemia

11. All the following statements regarding drug-drug interactions are true EXCEPT

(A) aspirin may increase the hypoprothrombinemic effect of dicumarol

(B) combining amphetamine and levothyroxine may cause cardiac tachyarrhythmias

(C) hydrochlorothiazide may increase the cardiac toxicity of digoxin

(D) cholestyramine enhances the hepatotoxicity of acetaminophen

(E) benztropine would increase the risk of urinary retention, paralytic ileus, and blurred vision associated with thioridazine

12. All the following statements are true about amphetamine EXCEPT that it

(A) releases catecholamines from central and peripheral adrenergic neurons

(B) may cause tachycardia, cardiac arrhythmias, and anginal pain

(C) is used in the treatment of narcolepsy

(D) is rapidly biotransformed by catechol-O-methyltransferase (COMT)

(E) can lead to toxic psychosis, hyperthermia, and hypertension

13. Which of the following is a selective inhibitor of monoamine oxidase B useful in the treatment of parkinsonism?

(A) Bromocriptine

(B) Carbidopa

(C) Deprenyl (selegiline)

(D) Phenelzine

(E) Tranylcypromine

14. The skeletal muscle relaxant that acts directly on the contractile mechanism of the muscle fibers is

(A) gallamine (Flaxedil)

(B) baclofen (Lioresal)

(C) pancuronium (Pavulon)

(D) cyclobenzaprine (Flexeril)

(E) dantrolene (Dantrium)

15. Select the enzyme that Metyrosine (Demser) inhibits.

(A) Tyrosine hydroxylase

(B) Acetylcholinesterase

(C) Catechol-O-methyltransferase

(D) Monoamine oxidase

(E) Carbonic anhydrase

16. The electrocardiogram of a patient who is receiving digitalis in the therapeutic dose range would be likely to show

(A) prolongation of the Q-T interval

(B) prolongation of the P-R interval

(C) symmetrical peaking of the T wave

(D) widening of the QRS complex

(E) none of the above

17. Cholestyramine (Questran) is a drug that is designed to lower blood cholesterol. Select the most appropriate mechanism of action for it.

(A) Decreases lipolysis in adipose tissue

(B) Decreases cholesterol synthesis at a rate-limiting step

(C) Increases the excretion of bile acids

(D) Decreases esterification of triglycerides in the liver and increases the activity of lipoprotein lipase

(E) Increases the activity of the lipid-clearing factor of heparin

18. Which of the following drugs is considered to be most effective in relieving and preventing ischemic episodes in patients with variant angina?

(A) Propranolol

(B) Nitroglycerine

(C) Sodium nitroprusside

(D) Nifedipine

(E) Isorbide dinitrate

19. What is the appropriate action for Coumarin derivatives?

(A) Inhibits thrombin and early coagulation steps

(B) Inhibits synthesis of prothrombin

(C) Inhibits platelet aggregation in vitro

(D) Activates plasminogen

(E) Binds the calcium ion cofactor in some coagulation steps

20. The synergistic effect from the combined use of a loop diuretic and a thiazide is due to reduction of sodium chloride reabsorption in the

(A) collecting duct

(B) ascending limb of the loop of Henle

(C) descending limb of the loop of Henle

(D) proximal tubule

(E) distal convoluted tubule

21. Idiopathic calcium urolithiasis can be treated by the administration of

(A) ethacrynic acid (Edecrin)

(B) triamterene (Dyrenium)

(C) furosemide (Lasix)

(D) hydrochlorothiazide (Hydrodiuril)

(E) bumetanide (Bumex)

22. For the diuretic agent Amiloride (Midamor), choose the anatomic site in the renal nephron where the principle action of the agent occurs.

(A) Glomerulus

(B) Proximal tubule

(C) Ascending limb of the loop of Henle

(D) Distal tubule

(E) Collecting duct

23. Drugs that bind to receptors in the plasma membrane and enhance levels of cyclic 3', 5'-adenosine monophosphate (cAMP) include all the following EXCEPT

(A) adrenocorticotropic hormone (ACTH)

(B) calcitonin

(C) isoproterenol

(D) hydrocortisone

(E) glucagon

24. True statements about testosterone include all the following EXCEPT

(A) it is biotransformed primarily in the liver

(B) it enhances the excretion of sodium and water

(C) it has a stimulatory effect on hematopoietic cells

(D) it attaches to a receptor on the X chromosome

(E) it is converted to an active metabolite, dihydrotestosterone (DHT)

25. A patient becomes markedly tetanic following a recent thyroidectomy. This symptom can be rapidly reversed by the administration of

(A) vitamin D

(B) calcitonin

(C) parathyroid hormone

(D) mithramycin

(E) calcium gluconate

PHYSIOLOGY I PRACTICE TEST
ANSWER SHEET

	ANS	CON			ANS	CON
1.				**14.**		
2.				**15.**		
3.				**16.**		
4.				**17.**		
5.				**18.**		
6.				**19.**		
7.				**20.**		
8.				**21.**		
9.				**22.**		
10.				**23.**		
11.				**24.**		
12.				**25.**		
13.						

CUT HERE

SEE PAGE **25** FOR INSTRUCTIONS
SEE PAGE **215** FOR ANSWERS

STUDY SUGGESTION

Intermittent review helps protect against forgetting and promotes the transfer of knowledge to long-term memory.

PHYSIOLOGY I

1. Secretion of pancreatic polypeptide is

(A) subsequent to its cleavage from proinsulin in the α cell
(B) a response to both vagal and β-adrenergic stimulation
(C) The stimulator of release of pancreatic enzymes in response to glucose
(D) inhibited by exercise
(E) none of the above

2. The graph below demonstrates diurnal variation in the plasma level of

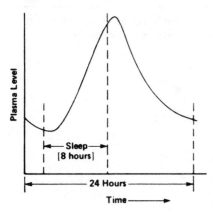

(A) thyroxine
(B) insulin
(C) parathyroid hormone
(D) cortisol
(E) estrogen

3. Insulin increases glucose uptake in all the following structures EXCEPT

(A) adipose tissue
(B) cardiac muscle
(C) skeletal muscle
(D) intestinal mucosa
(E) the uterus

4 - 6. For each hormone listed below, select the statement that best describes its mechanism of action.

(A) Binds to cell surface receptors and stimulates production of cyclic nucleotides in the cytoplasm
(B) Interacts with a cytoplasmic receptor, then localizes in the nucleus and directs protein and nucleotide synthesis
(C) Binds to cell surface receptors and then activates intracellular processes by a mediator other than cyclic nucleotides
(D) Interacts with a cytoplasmic receptor, then localizes in mito-chondria and directs oxidative metabolism
(E) None of the above

4. 1,25-Dihydroxycholecalciferol

5. Thyrotropin-releasing hormone

6. Cortisol

7. The largest portion of the arterial pressure generated during systole is dissipated at which of the following locations in the vascular tree?

(A) Aortic arch
(B) Aortic-arterial juncture
(C) Arterial-arteriolar juncture
(D) Arteriolar-capillary juncture
(E) Capillary-venular juncture

8. If the concentration of a substance within capillary blood decreases linearly along the length of a capillary, which of the following statements regarding its movement from capillary blood to interstitial fluid is correct?

(A) It will increase if capillary flow increases

(B) It will increase if its plasma concentration increases

(C) It will decrease if plasma oncotic pressure decreases

(D) Its rate is inversely related to molecular size

(E) None of the above

9. Cerebral blood flow is influenced by all the following EXCEPT

(A) viscosity of the blood

(B) P_{O_2} of lhe arterial blood

(C) cerebrospinal fluid pressure

(D) pH of the interstitial fluid of the brain

(E) vasomotor reflexes

10. Which of the following cardiac arrhythmias is LEAST likely to produce a change in the appearance of the QRS complex?

(A) First-degree heart block

(B) Second-degree heart block

(C) Third-degree heart block

(D) Atrial fibrillation

(E) Preventricular contraction

---

11 - 13. The tracing shown below represents a normal jugular venous pulse. For each of the following statements, select the lettered point that it best describes.

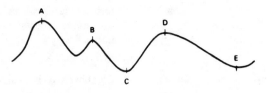

11. Becomes greatly amplified ("cannon wave") in patients with tricuspid stenosis

12. Increases in patients with tricuspid insufficiency

13. Is useful in distinguishing premature atrial contractions from premature ventricular contractions

14. At which point on the pressure volume curve illustrated below is the afterload on the heart the greatest?

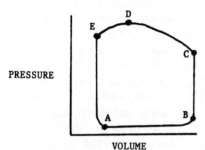

PRESSURE

VOLUME

(A) A

(B) B

(C) C

(D) D

(E) E

15. Which of the following statements about the third heart sound (S3) is correct?

(A) It is usually diminished in congestive heart failure

(B) It is produced by turbulence during rapid ventricular filling in the early diastole

(C) It is produced by turbulence following atrial contraction

(D) It is often associated with the "floppy" mitral valve syndrome

(E) It is produced by flow through the patent foramen ovale

16. Peripheral and central chemoreceptors may both contribute to the increased ventilation that occurs as a result of

(A) a decrease in arterial oxygen content

(B) a decrease in arterial blood pressure

(C) an increase in arterial carbon dioxide tension

(D) a decrease in arterial oxygen tension

(E) an increase in arterial pH

17 - 19. For each situation described below, select the combination of arterial blood pH and P_{CO_2} with which it is most likely to be associated.

(A) Increased pH, increased P_{CO_2}

(B) Increased pH, decreased P_{CO_2}

(C) Decreased pH, decreased P_{CO_2}

(D) Decreased pH, increased P_{CO_2}

(E) Normal pH, decreased P_{CO_2}

17. Suddenly increased respiratory rate, unchanged tidal volume

18. Living at a high altitude

19. Metabolic alkalosis

20. During quiet breathing, at the start of inspiration the intrapleural pressure is about -4 mmHg (relative to atmospheric pressure.) As inspiration proceeds, intrapleural pressure reaches approximately

(A) -8 mmHg

(B) -1 mmHg

(C) 0 mmHg

(D) + 1 mmHg

(E) + 8 mmHg

21. An increase in the concentration of plasma potassium causes an increase in

(A) release of renin

(B) secretion of aldosterone

(C) secretion of ADH

(D) release of natriuretic hormone

(E) production of angiotension II

22. Patient Y has a Pa_{CO_2} of 30 mmHg and a plasma bicarbonate concentration of 33 mmol/L. What is her concentration of plasma hydrogen ion (pH)?

(A) 18 nmol/L; pH = 7.75

(B) 28 nmol/L; pH = 7.56

(C) 33 nmol/L; pH = 7.49

(D) 40 nmol/L; pH = 7.40

(E) 48 nmol/L; pH = 7.32

23. Chronic administration of antacids and maintenance of a gastric pH that is about 7 would cause gastrin levels to

(A) decrease

(B) increase

(C) decrease, then subsequently increase

(D) increase, then decrease

(E) remain unchanged

24. All the following are correct statements about pancreatic exocrine secretion EXCEPT

(A) bicarbonate-rich fluid is secreted by ductal epithelial cells in response to secretin

(B) secretion of enzymes by acinar cells occurs in response to cholecystokinin

(C) vagotomy augments secretion of enzymes after a meal

(D) secretin and cholecystokinin both act via formation of cyclic nucleotide second messengers

(E) gastrin stimulates both enzyme and bicarbonate secretion

25. Pharmacologic blockade of histamine H_2 receptors in the gastric mucosa

(A) inhibits both gastrin-induced and vagally mediated secretion of acid

(B) inhibits gastrin-induced but not vagally mediated secretion of acid

(C) has no effect on either gastrin-induced or vagally mediated secretion of acid

(D) prevents activation of adenyl cyclase by gastrin

(E) causes an increase in potassium transport by gastric parietal (oxyntic) cells

PHYSIOLOGY II PRACTICE TEST
ANSWER SHEET

CUT HERE

	ANS	CON
1.		
2.		
3.		
4.		
5.		
6.		
7.		
8.		
9.		
10.		
11.		
12.		
13.		

	ANS	CON
14.		
15.		
16.		
17.		
18.		
19.		
20.		
21.		
22.		
23.		
24.		
25.		

SEE PAGE 25 FOR INSTRUCTIONS
SEE PAGE 216 FOR ANSWERS

STUDY SUGGESTION

Understanding increases memory retention and recall and leads to better problem solving. As you study, be sure that you really understand the material.

PHYSIOLOGY II

1. In a normal pregnancy, human chorionic gonadotropin (hCG) prevents the involution of the corpus luteum that normally occurs at the end of the menstrual cycle. Which of the curves shown below approximates the level of this hormone during pregnancy?

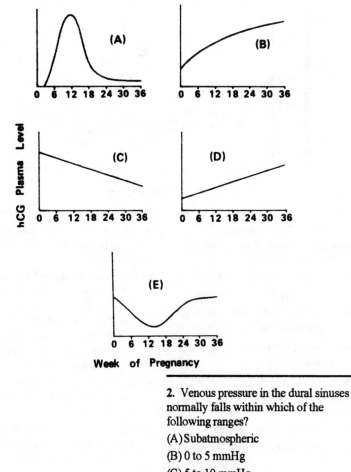

(A) A

(B) B

(C) C

(D) D

(E) E

2. Venous pressure in the dural sinuses normally falls within which of the following ranges?

(A) Subatmospheric

(B) 0 to 5 mmHg

(C) 5 to 10 mmHg

(D) 10 to 20 mmHg

(E) Greater than 20 mmHg

3. A normal dog receives an intravenous injection of pure crystalline insulin without glucose at time zero. Select the lettered curve on the graph that best represents the blood glucose pattern of the dog

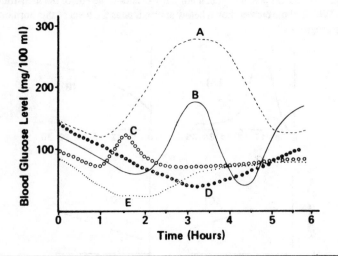

4. All the following statements concerning normal human pancreatic juice are true EXCEPT

(A) its pH is approximately 8.0

(B) it has a high bicarbonate content

(C) over 1000 ml are secreted per day

(D) it contains cholesterol esterase

(E) its secretion is primarily under neural control

5. In a nerve, the magnitude of the action potential overshoot is normally a function of the

(A) magnitude of the stimulus

(B) intracellular potassium concentration

(C) extracellular sodium concentration

(D) resting membrane potential

(E) diameter of the axon

6. The pH of the tubular fluid in the distal nephron can be lower than that in the proximal tubule because

(A) a greater sodium gradient can be established across the wall of the distal nephron than across the wall of the proximal tubule.

(B) more buffer is present in the tubular fluid of the distal nephron than in the proximal tubule

(C) more hydrogen ion is secreted into the distal nephron than into the proximal tubule

(D) the tight border of the distal nephron contains more carbonic anhydrase than that of the proximal tubule

(E) the tight junctions of the distal nephron are less leaky to solute than those of the proximal tubule

7. Which of the following statements regarding the flow of blood through the vascular bed pictured below (the numbers are the radii) is true?

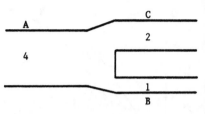

(A) The resistance of vessel C is two times the resistance of vessel A

(B) The resistance of vessel C is eight times the resistance of vessel A

(C) The flow through vessel C is twice the   flow through vessel B

(D) The flow through vessel C is four times the flow through vessel B

(E) None of the above

8. Peristaltic waves in the small intestine are characterized by which of the following statements?

(A) They are controlled primarily by extrinsic innervation

(B) They involve simultaneous contraction of the circular and longitudinal muscles

(C) They occur in response to distention of the wall

(D) They are preceded by increased fluid secretion by the intestinal mucosa

(E) None of the above

9. Citrate is a useful anticoagulant because of its ability to

(A) buffer basic groups of coagulation factors

(B) bind factor XII

(C) bind vitamin K

(D) chelate calcium

(E) be slowly metabolized

10. The greatest benefit derived from administering a positive inotropic drug to a patient in heart failure results from

(A) a reduction in heart rate

(B) a reduction in heart size

(C) an increase in contractile force

(D) an increase in wall thickness

(E) an increase in cardiac excitability

11. If the QRS complex is positive in lead II and negative in lead III, the mean electrical axis (MEA) is between

(A) –30 and +30

(B) +30 and +60

(C) +60 and +90

(D) +90 and +120

(E) +120 and +150

12. A patient is on a ventilator adjusted for a tidal volume of 1 L at a frequency of 10/min. If the patient's anatomical dead space is 200 ml and the machine's dead space 50 ml, the alveolar ventilation is

(A) 10 L/min

(B) 8 . 5 L/min

(C) 7 . 5 L/min

(D) 5 L/min

(E) not determinable from the information given

13. The figure shown below indicates the relation between myocardial fiber length and left ventricular stroke work. The solid curve, which indicates the normal response of the heart to a work load, represents Starling's law of the heart. The dotted line indicates the response of a normal heart when something has been superimposed to alter the heart's response. On the basis of Starling's law, the dotted line could indicate

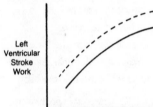

Left Ventricular Stroke Work

Left Ventricular End-Diastolic Fiber Length

(A) cardiac depression owing to hypoxia

(B) catecholamine response

(C) acetylcholine response

(D) congestive heart failure

(E) myocardial infarction

14. Injection of thyroid hormone into a normal laboratory animal will produce all the following effects EXCEPT

(A) an increase in the rate of oxygen consumption

(B) an increase in the rate of muscle protein synthesis

(C) an increase in the need for vitamins

(D) a decrease in the plasma concentration of cholesterol

(E) a decrease in the rate of lipolysis

15. Select the oxyhemoglobin dissociation curve that it is most likely to be associated with blood with a Pa_{CO_2} above normal.

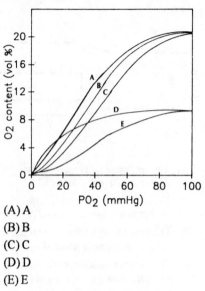

(A) A

(B) B

(C) C

(D) D

(E) E

16. Administration of pharmacologic doses of aldosterone to a dog will have which of the following effects upon blood pressure (BP), body weight (BW), and plasma potassium (PP) levels?

(Inc = Increased, Dec = Decreased)

	BP	BW	PP
(A)	Inc	Dec	Inc
(B)	Inc	Inc	Dec
(C)	Inc	Dec	Dec
(D)	Dec	Inc	Dec
(E)	Dec	Dec	Inc

17. The figures shown below depict the relationship of a substance's excretion rate (UV) and plasma clearance (UV/P) to its plasma concentration (U = urinary concentration, V = urinary flow rate, and P = plasma concentration). Based on these data, it can be seen that the substance is

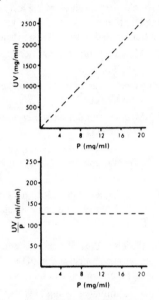

P (mq/ml)

P (mg/ml)

(A) not excreted in urine in proportion to its plasma concentration

(B) excreted in urine at a rate inversely proportional to its plasma concentration

(C) excreted in urine at a rate independent of its plasma concentration

(D) cleared from the body at a rate that decreases as its plasma concentration increases

(E) cleared from the body independently of its plasma concentration

18. The following measurements are obtained from a patient; PAH clearance = 750 ml/min; plasma creatinine concentration = 0.8 mg/100 ml; urinary creatinine concentration = 66 mg/100 ml; urinary excretion = 2 ml/min; plasma glucose concentration = 120 mg/100 ml.

What is the patient's filtration fraction?

(A) 0.18

(B) 0.20

(C) 0.22

(D) 0.24

(E) 0.26

19. The emptying rate of the stomach is regulated by hormonal and neural mechanisms that respond to both chemical and mechanical stimuli. The rate of gastric emtpying is influenced by all the following factors EXCEPT

(A) carbohydrate in gastric contents

(B) secretion of gastrin by antral G cells

(C) distention of the duodenal contents

(D) osmolarity of duodenal contents

(E) acidity of chyme entering the duodenum

20. The pancreas has both an endocrine and an exocrine function. The nonhormonal substances released by the pancreas serve all the following functions EXCEPT

(A) neutralizing the acid that enters the duodenum

(B) breaking down carbohydrate bonds

(C) breaking down lipids

(D) breaking down proteins

(E) increasein trypsin activity

21. Which one of the following will most likely cause body temperature to remain above normal?

(A) A decrease in the amount of blood flowing to the skin

(B) An increase in the intensity of exercise

(C) An increase in the set point of the thermoregulatory system

(D) An increase in production of thyroxine

(E) A decrease in the amount of evaporative water loss

22. The myotatic stretch reflex utilizes the smallest number of neurons of any cord reflex. Stretch of a muscle spindle causes all the following events EXCEPT

(A) excitation of receptors

(B) excitation of motor nerves

(C) transmission of impulses to anterior motor neurons

(D) a static as well as dynamic reflex

(E) relaxation of muscle

23. All the following statements about the eye are true EXCEPT that the

(A) focal point of hyperopic eye is behind the retina

(B) focal point of a myopic eye is in front of the retina

(C) focal point of an emmetropic eye is on the retina

(D) vision in a myopic eye can be corrected by use of a biconvex lens

(E) ciliary muscle is relaxed in an emmetropic eye focusing on an object 40 feet away

24. Two healthy women with identical tidal volumes and respiratory rates are subjected to spirometry and blood gas measurements. Subject A doubles her tidal volume and decreases her respiratory rate to one-half of baseline. Subject B decreases her tidal volume to one-half of baseline and doubles her respiratory rate. Which of the following statements about the resulting alveolar ventilation in the two women is true?

(A) Alveolar ventilation is unchanged in both subjects

(B) Alveolar ventilation increases in both subjects

(C) Alveolar ventilation decreases in both subjects

(D) Alveolar ventilation increases in subject A and decreases in subject B

(E) Alveolar ventilation decreases in subject A and increases in subject B

25. Which of the following statements about impulse transmission in the normal myoneural junction is true?

(A) It is stimulated by high levels of cholinesterase

(B) It is associated with an influx of potassium ions through the muscle membrane

(C) It is depressed by abnormally low levels of magnesium

(D) It is unaffected by extremely high rates of stimulation of the nerve fiber

(E) It is dependent upon the amount of acetylcholine released at the end-plate

Chapter 6

Course by Course

This chapter looks at each of the basic science subjects and suggests ways to review and to integrate across subjects.

OVERVIEW The USMLE covers subjects traditionally presented at most medical schools in seven basic science courses: Anatomy, Behavioral Science, Biochemistry, Microbiology, Pathology, Pharmacology, and Physiology. While much of the exam is based upon questions that are derived from individual subjects, the trend – indeed, the intent of the National Board – is to increase the proportion of questions that are integrative or cross-disciplinary. Thus, you should make every effort during your review to look for the relationships between details and concepts of one subject with others. This is not an easy thing to do but the suggestions following will help you become more integrative in your approach to review. In addition, the USMLE emphasizes clinically relevant basic science material: "Appproximately half of the items begin with a description of a clinical situation and require examinees to identify the cause of patient findings, to predict additional findings, or to specify the next step in patient cure, based on knowledge of basic science contents and principles." [1]

Review two subjects at the same time so that you are forced to think about how the facts and concepts of each are

---

[1] Swanson, D.B., Case, S.M. Melnick, D.E., & Volle, R.I. (1992) Impact of the USMLE Step 1. on Teaching and Learning of the Basic Biomedical Sciences. Academic Medicine, 67, 553-556.

related to each other. After the first two subjects, always review one new subject along with a subject previously reviewed. In this way, you help protect against forgetting material studied early in your review program.

Use a **systems approach** to organize your review so that you have a common basis for your study. For example, begin with the cardiovascular system, then the respiratory system, etc. The order in which you look at the various systems is not particularly important, but try to be consistent as you proceed from subject to subject.

Pick one **"anatomical" subject and one "functional" subject** when choosing the two subjects for study. By doing this, you will be able to continuously relate structure and function as you review. Identifying these kinds of relationships as you go along will greatly improve your remembering the information. However, be sure also to follow the guidelines discussed in Chapter 7 when you are making your schedule of subjects for review.

Construct tables that relate two subjects, for example, anatomy and physiology, and leave room to add others as your review progresses (pathology and pharmacology, for example). Making such tables is a form of active learning that will enhance your remembering of the material and also will permit quick and effective integrative review during the coming weeks before the board examination.

Pick a few disease states such as hypertension, diabetes mellitus, or fever and integrate the details and concepts of each subject area into your understanding of the disease. Construct tables and diagrams that summarize the information as you review each subject. Use any functional or structural changes that occur as a result of the disease to further your understanding of basic concepts. For example, list several functional changes that occur as a result of a chronic elevation in systemic arterial blood pressure. For each change, describe the underlying mechanisms that responded to the high blood pressure and led to the change. Do this type of analysis from the perspective of each course or subject. Put your analysis into a table for future review.

INTEGRATIVE REVIEW

1. Review two subjects simultaneously.
2. Use functional concepts as a framework for remembering structure.
3. Construct a table of facts and concepts that relates the two subjects at various levels of organization.
4. Use well-known diseases as a basis for understanding function.

EACH SUBJECT and DIABETES

In subsequent sections of this chapter, as an example, we will consider one disease, diabetes mellitus, and list a few points for analysis from the perspective of each specific subject. These special guidelines are in a shaded box such as this one under each course heading.

ANATOMY

Embryology
Histology
Gross Anatomy: Thorax
Gross Anatomy: Abdomen
Gross Anatomy: Pelvis
Gross Anatomy: Head and Neck
Gross Anatomy: Extremities and Back
Neuroanatomy

Anatomy is a course of details. As a result, you probably were inclined to study anatomy by memorizing the names and locations of structures. In many schools, the function of each structure or structural system is also taught but usually with little attention to the conceptual basis of the function. Since rote memorization of names, locations, and functions is not conducive to long-term remembering, you will probably have to devote quite a lot of time to your review of anatomy and its subdivisions.

One means of achieving an integrative approach to Anatomy is to review Embryology, Histology, Gross Anatomy, **and** Physiology together. Approach each topic by first considering the gross and histological structure, the embryology, and finally the function. Also, keep in mind that if you know the anatomy and function of one part of the body, you can rely on many parallels with other parts of the body. For example, the upper and lower extremities have much structure and function in common.

ANATOMY and DIABETES

- structure of the pancreas   - exocrine versus endocrine
- histology of the pancreas   - structure of the kidneys
- structure of blood vessels   - structure of membranes

BEHAVIORAL SCIENCE

Biological Correlates , Behavioral Genetics, Behavior & Personality, Learning & Change, Life-Span Development, Communication & Interaction, Group Processes, Family & Community, Sociocultural Patterns, Ecology & Disease, Health Care Systems, Statistics & Design

Behavioral Science, as presented in this book, is a conglomerate of somewhat diverse subjects. It includes the usual components of behavioral science as well as topics that are often taught in other courses. For example, we include epidemiology, biostatistics, and experimental design within this subject. In addition, some sociological subjects – aging and development, health care delivery systems, and aspects of medical practice – are also found here. When you organize your review, look for these topics within the framework of your own school's curriculum.

As for Anatomy, constructing tables is a very useful review tool. However, much of the information in the Behavioral Science category is conceptual in nature and requires you to consider processes and relationships. As you make tables of information for this subject, write brief summaries of each topic. Make sure you **understand** the concepts and are not merely describing or defining them.

BEHAVIORAL SCIENCE and DIABETES

- behavioral effects of living with diabetes on a child
- life expectancy and quality of life with the disease
- prevalence of the disease in racial groups, or by sex
- cost of care for the disease; impact on the poor
- design of a study of a new oral hypoglycemic
- family participation in required dietary restrictions

BIOCHEMISTRY

Amino Acids, Proteins, and Enzymes
Nucleic Acids
Carbohydrates and Lipids
Vitamins and Hormones
Membranes and Cell Structure
Metabolism

BIOCHEMISTRY is somewhat similar to Anatomy in that it contains a large number of details that must simply be memorized. However, coupled with these facts are many complex processes and pathways, the details of which must be understood as well as remembered. Moreover, while most of you learned Biochemistry more or less in isolation from the other basic medical sciences, its content obviously represents the molecular groundwork of physiology, pathology, pharmacology, etc.

To integrate your approach to Biochemistry, you might wish to review it in conjunction with Pharmacology (or Physiology). For example, when you review energy metabolism, consider it not only from the level of cellular metabolism and enzymes (biochemistry) but also as total body energy, caloric intake, heat production and loss, fever, antipyretics, metabolic poisons and antidotes, etc.

BIOCHEMISTRY and DIABETES
- structure of insulin, glucagon, and amino acids
- protein synthesis
- DNA/RNA structure and function
- carbohydrate metabolism
- structure of glucose, glycogen, etc.
- membrane structure/function, glucose transport

MICROBIOLOGY

Virology
Bacteriology
Physiology
Rickettsiae, Chlamydiae, and Mycoplasmas
Mycology
Parasitology
Immunology

Pay attention to the names, characteristics, and taxonomic classification of microorganisms as well as to their physiology. In addition, consider mechanisms of disease, transmission, virulence, ecology, and treatment.

This subject lends itself to summarizing in tables of information. Group organisms by taxonomic classification, physiology, pathogenicity, etc.

As you consider diseases caused by microorganisms, review anatomy, physiology, pathology, and pharmacology of affected tissues, organs, and systems. Also, don't forget topics like toxins, sterilization and disinfection, bacteriophages, and growth and cultivation of bacteria.

MICROBIOLOGY and DIABETES

- (Immunology); antigens, antibodies and insulin
- resistance to infection
- bacterial/viral infections and diabetes
- antibiotics and microbial metabolism and physiology

PATHOLOGY

General Pathology
Hematology
Cardiovascular System
Respiratory System
Gastrointestinal System
Endocrine System
Genitourinary System
Nervous System
Musculoskeletal System
Skin and Breast

This subject represents anatomy and histology revisited. When studying pathology, incorporate a general review of structure of tissues and organs. As you review the normal structure don't forget to consider function.

First review the normal structure (and function) and then consider the pathological changes. Add a pathology column to your review tables. Don't forget concepts and mechanisms when studying pathology. In addition to organ systems pathology, review general pathology, which includes such topics as cell injury, inflammation, genetics, immunopathology, neoplasia, and regeneration and repair.

PATHOLOGY and DIABETES

- pancreatic islets; hyalinization and fibrosis
- secondary lesions with diabetes
- mechanisms of gangrene and ulcers
- genetic influences
- obesity
- infections

PHARMACOLOGY

General Principles
Chemotherapy
Toxicology
Central Nervous System
Autonomic Nervous System
Cardiovascular System
Renal System
Endocrine System

Pharmacology is the study of how drugs affect physiology. Thus, you may wish to review these two subjects simultaneously. As you consider the heart, for example, review the physiology of cardiac functioning along with the mechanisms and effects of autonomic drugs or cardiac glycosides.

Make a column for pharmacology on your review tables to help you think about tissues, organs, and systems in an integrative, cross-disciplinary manner. Also, don't forget topics like drug absorption, distribution, metabolism, and excretion. Dose-response relationships and binding processes are also important.

PHARMACOLOGY and DIABETES

- use of hormones as drugs; replacement therapy
- blood levels, clearance, pharmacokinetics
- concept of receptors; agonists/antagonists
- oral hypoglycemics
- antibiotics

PHYSIOLOGY

Metabolism and Endocrinology
Cardiovascular System: Vascular
Cardiovascular System: Heart
Respiratory System
Renal and Acid-Base Physiology
Gastrointestinal System
Neurophysiology
Cellular Physiology

The subject of physiology like the others contains both details (facts) to be remembered and concepts to be understood and used in problem solving. As with the other subjects, your approach to learning (reviewing) must be different for the two kinds of information. Commit the details to memory so that you can recall them (not just recognize them) by repeatedly writing, discussing, or naming them. Enter these details into your summary tables. The conceptual material must be understood. This requires that you think about the concept, diagram it, write a summary, explain it to someone else, play with it, use it , etc. Finally, when you can recall the facts and the concepts are a "part of you," practice solving problems.

PHYSIOLOGY and DIABETES

- function of hormones, types, receptor mechanisms
- pancreatic function, control of insulin and glucagon
- carbohydrate metabolism and control
- control of hunger and thirst
- kidney function; filtration, reabsorption, secretion
- renal handling of glucose
- energy balance, control of body weight; temperature

Chapter 7

Designing a Study Plan

This chapter describes how to get organized and develop a study plan.

START NOW As you learned in Chapter 2, cramming is not a very good way to prepare for a comprehensive, integrative examination. Instead, make a complete, realistic study schedule that follows a regular, even pace over several weeks. Scheduling your time is very important. We have found over the years that the strongest students always have a plan of study for their courses and for review for major exams. Devising and maintaining a realistic study/review schedule is the best route to success on the USMLE.

Your schedule should take into account your present commitments – such as courses you are taking and their exams, holidays, planned vacations, family occasions, and other known time commitments – as well as the review time you need for the board exam. So start now and use the following guidelines to make up a realistic and complete study/review calendar for yourself for the next few weeks or months for your USMLE.

CONSTRUCTION OF YOUR PLAN In this section you will learn to construct a review program and write out a calendar to follow over the weeks you plan to study for the USMLE.

> **SET ASIDE TWO HOURS AND CONSTRUCT
> YOUR PLAN FOR REVIEW**

FIVE STEPS FOR CONSTRUCTING AND IMPLEMENTING A STUDY PLAN

Step One: Decide how many weeks you will need for your review program.

Step Two: Determine and enter each of your known commitments into the weekly calendar.

Step Three: Calculate how much total time you will have for reviewing for the USMLE and then divide that time among the seven basic science subjects.

Step Four: Give yourself a quiz at least once each week during your review program.

Step Five: Adjust your calendar based on the results of your self-evaluations and whether or not you are meeting your goals.

Constructing your own review program is the most important part of this plan for studying for the USMLE. If you do not have a plan, you will not be able to study efficiently, you may not be able to cover all of the materials you should, and you will increase your anxiety level because you will never be quite sure how you are progressing. Please make a plan. To do so properly will require only one or two hours. You should choose a time when you will not be interrupted and will have sufficient time to complete your planning. It is time well spent that will save you considerable worry and frustration as the USMLE draws near.

The first three steps in constructing your review plan need to be done now. The last two steps are repeated during the upcoming weeks as you follow your plan. It is all very easy to do – just follow the outline below:

Step One: Decide how many weeks you will need for your review program.

We recommend that you begin your review as early as possible. If you are currently enrolled in second-year courses, you should begin now with a few hours each week devoted to the material from first-year courses. However, you may review for any amount of time that seems appropriate for your needs. Whatever amount of time you choose, make your choice and sit right down to construct your plan for review.

You can decide how many weeks you need by estimating how many hours you must spend on each course and by determining how much *reviewing* time you will have each week. However, the longer the duration of your review program, the better prepared you will be for the USMLE. In other words, it is much better to review 10 hours each week for 20 weeks than 20 hours per week for 10 weeks even though the total review time is 200 hours in both cases (see Chapter 2).

HOW MUCH TIME IS NEEDED TO SUCCESSFULLY PREPARE FOR STEP 1?

THIS DEPENDS UPON:

—HOW WELL YOU WANT TO DO

> **Merely Pass**
> **Average**
> **Excel** (If seeking competitive residency)

—YOUR GRADES IN MEDICAL SCHOOL

> Students who have **failed** courses tend to have
>   more trouble passing the board exam
> **Marginal** students have more trouble
> **Average** students tend to be average
> **Honors** students tend to do well

—YOUR STUDY METHOD IN MEDICAL SCHOOL

> **Crammers** tend to be disappointed in their
>   scores
> **Active learners** who made good summaries
>   tend to do better

—YOUR UNDERSTANDING OF THE MATERIAL INITIALLY

> Don't expect to remember if you didn't really under-
>   stand what you were learning in the first place

—HOW WELL YOU LEARNED MATERIAL IN THE FIRST PLACE

> Material you understand but have only studied lightly
>   or not recently will need to be reviewed

It is unlikely that any enrolled student will be able to devote more than 350 total hours to reviewing for the USMLE, even if review is initiated at the beginning of second year and full use is made of vacation time. This means that, on average, each basic science can be given about 50 hours. A more realistic schedule includes about 210 hours total review time or an average of 30 hours per subject. Once you have decided upon the duration of your review program, purchase a calendar.

Step Two: Determine and enter each of your known commitments into the weekly calendar.

Now enter into your calendar all your known commitments for the weeks you have chosen for review. Time commitments may be thought of as belonging to one of five categories:

Categories of Commitments

1. Academic (classes, exams, study, etc.)
2. Life Maintenance (sleep, eating, shopping, etc.)
3. Social (phone calls, birthdays, parties, etc.)
4. Leisure (movies, sports, TV, etc.)
5. Other (travel, religious, etc.)

When you begin to enter your commitments into your calendar, take your time, be thoughtful, and be as complete as possible. It is very important that you enter everything you are committed to doing during the weeks of your review plan. First, look over the general time commitments listed on the next page and try to think of others that apply to your life. As you think of any, categorize them and then write them into the appropriate spot in the list.

GENERAL TIME COMMITMENTS

Academic

attending classes	examinations
laboratories	reports
seminars	studying

_____   _____

_____   _____

Life Maintenance

exercise	lunch
dinner	sleep
breakfast	laundry
relaxation	legal matters
food shopping	banking
paying bills	

_____   _____

Social

dates	telephoning
wedding	birthdays
parties	

_____   _____

Leisure

holidays	trips
vacation	sports
movies	television

_____   _____

Other

travel to school	moving
religious observance	

_____   _____

_____   _____

Once you have all the general time commitments listed, enter your specific commitments into your calendar. Enter your academic commitments first since these are the least flexible. Continue to fill in your calendar, entering commitments in the order presented in the list above. Enter them day by day, assigning time in one-hour blocks. Be sure to enter everything and be generous in assigning time to your commitments. Check your calendar several times to ensure that you didn't forget anything. Be sure to include time for meals, sleep, play, and study for the courses you are currently taking. Use the list of General Time Commitments to jog your memory.

> **Step Three:** Calculate how much total time you will have for reviewing for the USMLE and then divide that time among the seven basic science subjects.

Having entered all your known commitments into your calendar, you are ready to assign review time. Proceed as follows:

1. Find the uncommitted times in your calendar and mark them with a red pen.

2. Select the hours that are appropriate for board preparation. You might discover, for example, that every Saturday morning (with the exception of weekends before exams in your courses) you can devote 2 hours to board preparation.

3. Count the total number of USMLE preparation hours and enter the total on **line 1** in the box on the next page. It is important not to overestimate how much time you can afford to devote to review. If you do so, you probably will not be able to keep to your schedule, will not complete your exam preparation, and may end up frustrated and anxious.

4. Calculate 20 percent of the total on **line 1** and enter the result on **line 2**. This will be deducted from the total to allow for commitments you didn't think of as well as for unexpected new commitments that come up from time to time.

5. Subtract the deductible hours from the total uncommitted hours and enter the result on **line 3**. This new number is a realistic total number of hours available to you for review during the course of your chosen plan.

You now must apportion your realistic total review time among the topics you need to review. As a first approximation of how much review time you will have for each course, divide the number on line 3 by 7 (for each of the basic science courses) and enter the result on **line 4**.

CALCULATION OF AVAILABLE REVIEW HOURS

1. **TOTAL USMLE REVIEW HOURS** ____

2. **THE DEDUCTIBLE (20%)** (___)

3. **TOTAL REALISTIC HOURS** ____

4. **APPROXIMATE TIME PER COURSE** ____

It is unlikely that you will need to spend the same amount of time on each subject. A better apportionment of your review time depends upon your ability to evaluate your relative need to review each subject. To make such an evaluation, follow the instructions for assigning review priorities provided in the table on the next page.

GUIDELINES FOR ASSIGNING REVIEW PRIORITIES

— Allot more time to the subjects with which you are <u>least</u> comfortable. (See page 10)

— Evaluate your proficiency in each of the basic sciences; identify which are your strengths and which are your weaknesses.

— Make an ordered list of the basic sciences that reflects your mastery of the subjects from worst to best. Assign a number (1 to 7) where 7 is the subject you know best and 1 is your worst subject.

— Also, within each subject, assign to each of the subtopics a number that reflects your proficiency from worst to best.

— Begin your review with the subjects that give you the greatest difficulty. Devote more time to topics within each subject that are weak ones for you.

— Don't waste time on topics with which you are comfortable, but don't neglect these areas entirely. A cursory review of these topics should suffice.

You may decide to assign only a little review time to some subjects or topics. For example, if you are taking Pharmacology during the Spring term while you are reviewing, you may wish to schedule only a small amount of time at the end of your review plan for a quick overview of the entire course. If the exams in such a course are not cumulative or your grades are marginal, you may require more review time.

SUBJECT RANKS AND APPORTIONED HOURS

SUBJECT	RANK	REVIEW HOURS	PRACTICE SCORES PRE	POST
Anatomy				
Behavioral Science				
Biochemistry				
Microbiology				
Pathology				
Pharmacology				
Physiology				
TOTAL				

The following series of tables can help you refine your apportionment of time within each subject. Based on the number of subtopics per subject, assign a number based upon your evaluation of your knowledge and preparedness. Rank them high to low for best to worst, then apportion the hours you gave to the main subject (in the table above) among its subtopics, giving the lowest numbered subtopics the greatest amount of review time. Space has also been provided for you to enter your scores on pre- and postreview practice tests in each subject and subtopic. These scores will further help you apportion your review hours.

SUBTOPIC RANKS AND APPORTIONED HOURS
ANATOMY

SUBJECT	RANK	REVIEW HOURS	PRACTICE SCORES PRE	POST
Embryology				
Histology				
Thorax				
Abdomen				
Pelvis				
Head & Neck				
Extremities; Back				
Neuroanatomy				
TOTAL				

(Assign ranks of 1 through 8)

SUBTOPIC RANKS AND APPORTIONED HOURS
BEHAVIORAL SCIENCE

SUBJECT	RANK	REVIEW HOURS	PRACTICE SCORES PRE	POST
Biological Correlates				
Behavioral Genetics				
Personality				
Learning				
Life Span				
Communication				
Group Processes				
Family & Community				
Sociocultural Patterns				
Ecology & Disease				
Health Care Systems				
Statistics & Design				
TOTAL				

(Assign ranks of 1 through 12)

SUBTOPIC RANKS AND APPORTIONED HOURS
BIOCHEMISTRY

SUBJECT	RANK	REVIEW HOURS	PRACTICE SCORES PRE	POST
Amino acids, Proteins				
Nucleic Acids				
Carbohydrates, Lipids				
Vitamins & Hormones				
Cell Structures				
Metabolism				
TOTAL				

(Assign ranks of 1 through 6)

SUBTOPIC RANKS AND APPORTIONED HOURS
MICROBIOLOGY

SUBJECT	RANK	REVIEW HOURS	PRACTICE SCORES PRE	POST
Virology				
Bacteriology				
Physiology				
Rickettsiae, etc.				
Mycology				
Parasitology				
Immunology				
TOTAL				

(Assign ranks of 1 through 7)

SUBTOPIC RANKS AND APPORTIONED HOURS
PATHOLOGY

SUBJECT	RANK	REVIEW HOURS	PRACTICE SCORES PRE	POST
General				
Hematology				
Cardiovascular				
Respiratory				
Gastrointestinal				
Endocrine				
Genitourinary				
Neural				
Musculoskeletal				
Skin & Breast				
TOTAL				

(Assign ranks of 1 through 10)

SUBTOPIC RANKS AND APPORTIONED HOURS
PHARMACOLOGY

SUBJECT	RANK	REVIEW HOURS	PRACTICE SCORES PRE	POST
General Principles	___	___	___	___
Chemotherapy	___	___	___	___
Toxicology	___	___	___	___
Central Nervous	___	___	___	___
Autonomic Nervous	___	___	___	___
Cardiovascular	___	___	___	___
Renal	___	___	___	___
Endocrine	___	___	___	___
TOTAL	___			

(Assign ranks of 1 through 8)

SUBTOPIC RANKS AND APPORTIONED HOURS
PHYSIOLOGY

SUBJECT	RANK	REVIEW HOURS	PRACTICE SCORES PRE	POST
Metabolism	___	___	___	___
Endocrinology	___	___	___	___
Vascular	___	___	___	___
Heart	___	___	___	___
Respiratory	___	___	___	___
Renal	___	___	___	___
Acid-Base	___	___	___	___
Gastrointestinal	___	___	___	___
Neurophysiology	___	___	___	___
Cellular	___	___	___	___
TOTAL	___			

(Assign ranks of 1 through 10)

Make certain that the total hours assigned to each course, topic by topic, are equal to the total hours assigned to each course in the **Subject Ranks and Apportioned Hours** table of the previous section.

You are now ready to actually assign specific days and hours to review each of the subjects and their subtopics. Remember, begin with the subject that you ranked first (your worst) and its subtopics with the lowest ranking. These are the areas where you need the most work.

You may want to work on two subjects in parallel. For example, if you study Physiology and Pathology together, you can study systems in both subjects simultaneously: cardiovascular physiology with cardiovascular pathology, endocrine physiology with endocrine pathology, and so on. This is a very effective way to integrate the sciences (see Chapter 6).

Turn to your calendar and write in the topics to be reviewed in each of the hours you have available for USMLE preparation.

> Use a **pencil** when entering items into your calendar; you will have to make adjustments later on based on the results of self-assessments.

Be sure to schedule at least **one hour each week for testing yourself** on your progress (see Step Four next). When you have finished filling in your schedule, you should have several hours (20%) free of any scheduled topic. Use these hours for topics that need more work than you first calculated or for other unforeseen needs.

Step Four: Give yourself a quiz at least once each week during your review program.

It is very important that you monitor your progress throughout your review program. To do this, you must take regular quizzes (one each week) in each of the subjects you are studying. As you progress through your review program, these weekly quizzes will indicate which topics you should assign to the "open" hours for extra review time.

Be sure to schedule your self-testing at logical points in your review each week. Use an hour to take a short quiz as you complete your review of each subtopic in a science and then analyze the results to determine where further review is needed. The PreTest® books published by McGraw-Hill, Inc., are organized by subtopics so that you can do this easily. Furthermore, we have prepared comprehensive quizzes in each subject for you which are presented in Chapter 5 along with complete instructions on how to use them.

Step Five: Adjust your calendar based on the results of your self-evaluations and whether or not you are meeting your goals.

Each week during your self-testing hour you should consider your entire review schedule and decide if you need to adjust it. On the basis of quiz results, you may decide to stop reviewing one topic and add time to another, add an additional topic to your schedule, schedule more quizzes, or alter the order in which you review subjects and topics. Be flexible. Remember you have spare time built into the calendar and you may use some of those hours if you need to.

Try however, to keep spare hours throughout the course of your review plan. As you progress through your schedule, use the spare hours and move everything up so that the extra hours are always ahead of you. You may become ill and not be able to study or you may just need to take a break from it all. Whatever the reason, those extra hours will be very useful as the USMLE draws near.

A Sample Review Schedule

On the following page, we have constructed a sample review schedule. It assumes the student needs (or has) 12 weeks for review. You, of course, may choose a longer or shorter length of time as dictated by your needs and other time constraints. As discussed at the beginning of this chapter, pick as long a duration of review as possible (20 weeks is better than 12 weeks but 12 is better than 4).

The sample plan assumes the following subject ranks for apportioning review hours:

Subject	Rank
Anatomy	1
Behavioral Science	7
Biochemistry	3
Microbiology	5
Pathology	4
Pharmacology	2
Physiology	6

As you can see, this hypothetical student's worst subjects are Anatomy and Pharmacology and the best are Behavioral Science and Physiology. Thus, in the review plan, the first subject studied is Anatomy but it is reviewed along with a strong subject, Physiology. Also, these subjects complement each other by allowing the integration of structure and function.

A SAMPLE 12-WEEK REVIEW SCHEDULE

WEEKS 1, 2, and 3
ANATOMY (weakest subject; rank 1)
PHYSIOLOGY (strong subject; rank 6)
Rationale: Start review with worst subject, Anatomy, and review it along with a strong subject, Physiology.

WEEKS 4 and 5
PHARMACOLOGY (weak subject; rank 2)
(PHYSIOLOGY) (6)
Rationale: Review next worst subject, Pharmacology, and couple it with a second review of Physiology.

WEEKS 6 and 7
BIOCHEMISTRY (weak subject; rank 3)
(PHARMACOLOGY) (2)
Rationale: Review Biochemistry next (ranks third) and couple it with a second look at Pharmacology. Could also consider appropriate Physiology topics that appear on the review table constructed in previous weeks.

WEEKS 8, 9, and 10
PATHOLOGY (good subject; rank 4)
(ANATOMY) (1)
Rationale: Spend 3 weeks reviewing Pathology, a large subject area, and also consider Anatomy for the second time.

WEEK 11
MICROBIOLOGY (strong subject; rank 5)
(BIOCHEMISTRY) (3)
Rationale: Microbiology is one of the stronger subjects so only a week near the end of the review program is sufficient. Also schedule a brief, second look at Biochemistry.

WEEK 12
BEHAVIORAL SCIENCE (strongest subject; rank 7)
Rationale: For the last week of the review program, go over your best subject, Behavioral Science. Study the summaries and integrative review tables developed throughout the entire review program. Work on any problem areas detected by the use of self-tests. Get plenty of sleep, plenty of exercise, and eat well this last week before the USMLE. Refrain from using alcohol. Relax a little. Go see a good movie or attend a concert. You are ready for the test.

STUDY SUGGESTION

As you study, try to anticipate what information will be included in each section of your review book.

As you review, identify (e.g., highlight) information that you did not remember, did not know, or are having difficulty understanding.

What decisions must be made to answer this question?

Which of the following is noted in Cushing's syndrome, a tumor-associated disease of the adrenal cortex.
      A. Decreased production of epinephrine
      B. Excessive production of epinephrine
      C. Excessive production of vasopressin
      D. Excessive production of cortisol
      E. Decreased production of cortisol

(See **Biochemistry: PreTest®**, 6th ed., #360, p. 150.)

Test-taking strategies are discussed in detail in the next chapter. See page 210 for a discussion of this question.

Chapter 8

Test-Taking Strategies

This chapter describes how you should prepare your-self physically and psychologically for the examination, and how to take it efficiently and effectively.

INTRODUCTION To maximize performance on multiple-choice examinations, it is important that you have a systematic and organized approach. Without such an approach, effective pacing and performance may be compromised. It also helps if you are well prepared physically and psychologically for the exam. The following suggestions should lead to optimal performance, given your level of preparation, and minimize the likelihood of careless errors.

BEFORE THE EXAM

Anxiety Most students experience a certain amount of anxiety when faced with major examinations. Some anxiety can actually be a good thing, since it helps you focus your attention, think carefully, and be on the alert for careless mistakes. However, if you tend to be so anxious during exams that your performance suffers, consider taking a short course in stress management or in relaxation training. Take the course well in advance of the actual exam so that you learn and practice the techniques. As with any skill, relaxing in the face of a challenging event requires lots of practice before it can be done efficiently and effectively.

Food Eat foods for energy and be sure not to choose ones likely to produce indigestion or other kinds of GI distress.

Exercise Try to get regular exercise during the weeks leading up to the exam. Exercise will keep your body in good physical shape, help you sleep better, and reduce anxiety. If you feel good physically, you will be able to perform better on the day of the USMLE. If you are not used to exercise, don't overdo it. Sore muscles and tendons are a distraction you don't need.

Sleep Try to get a good night's sleep before the exam. If you tend to be the type who has difficulty sleeping the night before an exam such as this, be certain that you get several good nights of sleep before the day-before-the-exam. This will minimize the fatigue effects of a poor night's sleep during the exam.

THE DAY OF THE EXAM

What to Take: Your registration materials, several sharpened #2 pencils, erasers, snacks (such as an apple, chocolate bar, or a sandwich), a small pillow, drinks, etc.

What Not to Take: Calculators, electronic wrist watches, etc. If you happen to have a cold, you must not take medications that cause drowsiness.

What to Wear: Be sure to wear comfortable, nonbinding clothes. You can't be sure what the temperature will be like in your testing center, so wear layers that can be put on or taken off to accommodate different temperatures. Being too hot can be fatiguing and being too cold can be equally uncomfortable and distracting.

How to Cope with Fatigue: During the breaks, you might take a short nap in your car (be sure to set an alarm). Some students have found that the exercise of a brisk walk or run helps reinvigorate them. Most examinees drink coffee or caffeinated soda. Do this only if you are used to the effects of caffeine.

> # HOW TO APPROACH THE EXAM ITSELF

There are four major components to performing optimally as you take this examination: **the basic mechanics, deductive reasoning, elimination strategies**, and **guessing strategies.** In addition, specific strategies by question types used in USMLE Step 1 are discussed.

1. The Basic Mechanics

The basic mechanics of taking the exam include approaches to sequence, filling in the answer form, and pacing, as well as several suggestions concerning how to read, understand, and answer each question. These can help you maximize efficiency in taking the exam.

Sequence Answer every question in sequence, even if you must guess (see Section 4 on Guessing Strategies). <u>Do not leave any blanks</u>. In other words, start with question 1 in each booklet and work through to the last question, filling in an answer for every question. A potential pitfall of skipping questions is that you run the risk of leaving blanks when time is called at the end of the exam. Scanning an almost-full answer form looking for blank spaces is a difficult perceptual task even when you have lots of time. Every blank on your answer form is a lost point on the exam, so be sure to get the possibility of every point by answering every question. Another benefit of answering questions as you encounter them is that, in the absence of firm knowledge, your first hunches are more likely to be right than second or third hunches. Finally, proceeding through the exam answering only the questions about which you are sure further wastes time since it requires reading questions twice (once when you decide you are not sure and once again when you retry).

Filling in the answer form Fill in the optically scanned answer form as you answer each question. Do not wait until the end of the exam to transfer answers from your booklet to the answer form. This is much too time-consuming and there is an increased likelihood of transcription errors: filling in answers in the wrong row. We have heard many "nightmare" stories from students who did not detect a transcription error until near the end of the exam and who then had to spend valuable time erasing and refilling in the boxes.

Pacing Pace yourself carefully. You will have an average of 50 to 60 seconds per question. Do not spend an excessive amount of time on any one question. This could limit your time for subsequent questions which, with adequate time, you could answer correctly. If you think you can figure out the answer, but it's taking too much time, guess and circle the question number and return to the question if time remains after you have completed the rest of the questions (see section on Guessing Strategies). Subsequent questions may help you focus your reasoning or recall pertinent information. Do not forget that some questions can be answered very quickly, in much less time than the average, while others are more difficult and require longer than average.

Pacing should be done on average not per question. Develop the habit of checking your watch every 30 questions to determine if your pacing needs to be modified. Clearly, if you have answered 30 questions in well under 30 minutes, you are pacing yourself effectively. However, if you have taken 35 to 40 minutes to complete 30 questions, you will need to speed up somewhat. Of course if you have just completed 30 lengthy questions, you can probably make up the time on subsequent shorter, more straightforward questions.

Changing answers DO NOT change an answer when reconsidering UNLESS you feel a higher degree of confidence about the new answer.

> If you experience the "AH HAAA!!! Now I get it" phenomenon, it is okay to change the answer.

Don't forget that first hunch answers are correct with a higher probability than second hunch answers. Do not let lack of confidence in yourself make you change answers.

> Do not let *"Gee, I probably didn't learn this well, so the right answer must be this answer that I've never heard of"* motivate answer changes.

Read each question very carefully Pay attention to key words and qualifiers (e.g., sometimes, always, most, not, etc.,).

Underline key words Underline or circle key words or parts of words in the question. This will help ensure that you don't lose track of important information as you reason through the question. Jot down relevant ideas, equations, etc., to help keep your thinking focused.

Anticipate answers When possible you should try to anticipate the answer to the question before reading the alternatives, since this will decrease the likelihood that the distractors (i.e., the incorrect alternatives) will actually distract you. It will also help you identify an inaccurate or inattentive reading of the question.

> If the alternatives don't make sense when you look at them, you probably misread the question.

Get a sense of the question After reading the question, to get a sense of the kind of information that will be relevant to the answer, scan all the alternatives. This helps you focus your thinking and approach the question in a systematic and logical manner.

Record your reaction Note your reaction to each alternative (next to the alternative letter) using the following codes:

Codes for reactions to alternatives

T   =   True statement
T? =   Possibly true: sounds plausible, but...
F   =   False statement
F? =   Possibly False: doesn't sound right, but...
?   =   No idea what this means

These codes are especially useful for students who consistently choose the wrong answer when they have narrowed the choice to two alternatives and to students who have low confidence in their knowledge. Most students merely put a slash (/) through alternatives that they have ruled out, and they leave options unmarked that are possibly correct or which they are uncertain about. This tactic can cause problems since it focuses attention on the doubt associated with particular alternatives, as opposed to the possible truth value (true or false).

The initial impression about the truth value of the statement (e.g., "well, that sounds plausible, but..." or "that doesn't sound right, but...") is more likely to be correct than subsequent impressions based on reasoning that is motivated primarily by the uncertainty.

It is more productive to consider why you think a statement sounds plausible (or unlikely) than to try to come up with reasons why your reasoning might be flawed. If you use the codes described above to help capture these initial reactions to alternatives, you can take advantage of first hunches and thus be able to focus subsequent reasoning more effectively. Everyone has these initial impressions, so it does **not** take any extra time to come up with them. The fraction of a second that it takes to record them next to each alternative can actually help focus your reasoning, thereby saving time overall.

The above strategy can also be applied to EXCEPT, LEAST, and NOT TRUE questions in the following manner:

Circle the words EXCEPT, LEAST, or NOT TRUE in the question and read the question without the circled word. Use the codes described above (T, T?, F, F?, ?) in the usual fashion. The lone "F" (if you can narrow the options) will be the answer.

This strategy prevents you from having to redefine your slashes as you tackle these question types, thereby preventing careless errors. If an alternative that is eliminated is merely slashed out (e.g., _A_), then the slash signifies "True" for EXCEPT/LEAST/NOT TRUE type questions but "False" for

BEST answer questions. For example, consider the following question:

> In addition to the vas deferens, structures normally found within the internal spermatic fascia of the spermatic cord include all the following EXCEPT the
> A. Deferential artery
> B. Ilioinguinal nerve
> C. Pampiniform plexus
> D. Testicular artery
> E. Testicular nerve
>
> [See **Anatomy PreTest® Self-Assessment and Review**, 6th ed., # 273, answer p. 142 (B)]

By crossing out the word, "EXCEPT," the question reads, "... structures normally found within the internal spermatic fascia of the spermatic cord include all the following." Now you can simply read each alternative and if the option is normally found within the region described, mark it with "T," if not, mark it with "F," and so on. The single alternative coded "F" will be the correct answer for any negatively phrased questions (EXCEPT, LEAST, NOT TRUE).

Read the entire question Read ALL the alternatives carefully before selecting an answer. Even when you are certain about your answer, read the other alternatives thoughtfully to cross check your reasoning.

On the next page is an example of how to apply all the techniques described above to a Best Answer question. Notice the underlining and circling of all key words in the question stem. Circle key information that may be overlooked and underline other key words.

For 2 weeks a 3-year-old child has experienced petechiae and bleeding of the gums. On examination, he is pale and his temperature is 39°C. This clinical picture is compatible with:

F   A. Chronic Lymphocytic Leukemia
T   B. Acute Lymphocytic Leukemia
F   C. Chronic Myelogenous Leukemia
F   D. Acute Myelogenous Leukemia
F   E. Infectious Mononucleosis

By scanning the collection of alternatives, it becomes clear that three decisions must be made in order to answer the question.

The first decision: Is this Leukemia (alternatives A - D) or Mononucleosis (E)? Since **bleeding gums** and **petechiae** are not symptoms of Mononucleosis, alternative (E) can be ruled out.

The second decision: Is this a Chronic (A and C) or an Acute (B and D) condition? Since the condition has only been evident for **2 weeks**, chronic conditions (A and C) are less likely.

The third decision: Is this Lymphocytic (A and B) or Myelogenous (C and D) Leukemia? Since Acute Lymphocytic Leukemia is most common in children, option "B" can be selected.

All these mechanisms will help you should you have time to reconsider your answer for a particular question. Without such markings, you waste time reconstructing your initial reasoning as opposed to reevaluating your reasoning.

A SUMMARY OF THE BASIC MECHANICS

Answer questions in order; don't skip
Fill in the answer form as you go
Pace yourself carefully
Do NOT change answers without good reason
Read each question very carefully
Underline key words
Anticipate answers to focus your thinking
Get a sense of the question; scan the options
Record your reactions (T, T?, F, F?, ?)
Read ALL the alternatives carefully

Simple Matching questions use a single alternative set (A, B, C,...Z) for more than one question (see Chapter 1). Therefore, it is not easy to apply the basic mechanics we just described whereby you record your reactions to the alternatives. However, you can mark your initial answer in the left margin as indicated below (A - E), and record "T," "F," and "?" next to it to keep track of your reasoning for each question. Don't forget that each alternative can be used once, more than once, or not at all.

For each disease listed below, select the virus most likely to be the causative agent.

A. Cytomegalovirus
B. Rotavirus
C. Varicella-zoster virus
D. Adenovirus
E. Papillomavirus

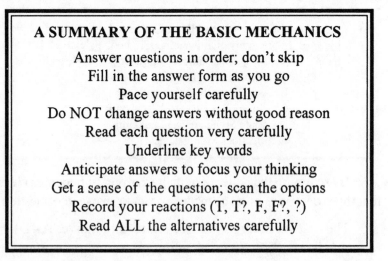

102. Chicken pox
103. Acute respiratory disease (ARD)
104. Human warts

(See **Microbiology: PreTest® Self-Assessment and Review**, 6th ed., # 102 - 104, answers p. 36.)

2. Deductive Reasoning

Deductive reasoning skills enable you to effectively narrow the options in the face of only partial knowledge. Applying these skills can improve chance performance and, hence, exam scores considerably. Students frequently fail to access all of their deductive reasoning skills when approaching multiple-choice exam questions. Instead they guess hastily on questions for which they feel their knowledge or understanding is weak or lacking altogether.

Every question, however, deserves a fair reading and a reasonable attempt. When you are uncertain about a question, use effective deductive reasoning skills to eliminate or narrow the options to improve chance performance. Below are some important recommendations on how to approach questions in the face of uncertainty.

Search for the ridiculous option(s) Multiple-choice questions often contain at least one alternative that is "off the wall." Be sure to eliminate such options before giving up on the question entirely and simply guessing. Try this question:

A 28-year-old menstruating woman appeared in the emergency room with the following signs and symptoms: fever, 104° F (40° C); wbc, 16,000/mm³; blood pressure, 90/65 mmHg; a scarlatina rash on her trunk, palms and soles; extreme fatigue; vomiting; and diarrhea. The most characteristic finding not yet revealed in the case just presented would be

A. Travel to Vermont
B. Recent exposure to rubella
C. A retained tampon
D. A meal of chicken in a fast-food restaurant
E. Heavy menstrual flow

(See **Microbiology: PreTest® Self-Assessment and Review**, 6th ed., # 171, answer p. 68.)

Alternatives A, B, and D can all be considered ridiculous options in this question. Alternative A is simply not relevant and can be eliminated immediately. While some of the symptoms of the patient may be consistent with rubella (B) and others with salmonella (D), neither of these conditions has anything to do with the fact that this woman is menstruating; even if you can't remember all the symptoms of the diseases, you can rule out both alternatives on the grounds that they simply have nothing to do with menstruation and are therefore "ridiculous." Don't forget that the questions are not designed to "lead you down the garden path" by presenting extraneous, misleading information. The answer is C.

Word roots Analyzing the roots of words can help you narrow the options. Consider the following question:

An agent is introduced into a growing bacterial colony and cell multiplication ceases. Removal of the agent, however, allows bacterial cell division to resume. This agent would be described as:

    A. A disinfectant
    B. A bacteriocide
    C. An antiseptic
    D. A bacteriostat
    E. A sterilizer

(See **Microbiology: PreTest® Self-Assessment and Review,** 5th ed., p. 69 for a discussion of this question.)

The root "cide" means to kill as in suicide, genocide, etc. The root "stat" means to stop. The correct answer to this question is D.

Consider all the information If information is given in the question stem, treat it as relevant to the selection of an alternative. The USMLE questions are not designed to mislead you but are meant to be straightforward.

> If information is given in the stem, treat it as relevant.

Every piece of information must be consistent with the correct alternative. Read the following rather lengthy example:

A 25-year-old woman is seen by her physician because of progressive dyspnea, fatigue, and syncope on exertion. She has no history of rheumatic fever or heart murmur. The patient was in excellent health until 6 months ago when her symptoms developed; they have since become progressively worse. Physical examination reveals a well-developed, well-nourished, acyanotic woman who experiences mild respiratory distress at rest. The jugular pulse reveals large alpha waves. There is a prominent right ventricular heave. A palpable pulmonic closure is present. A grade III/VI systolic ejection murmur is heard at the left second intercostal space. A grade I/IV blowing, holosystolic murmur is also noted at the lower left sternal border. The pulmonic closure is loud but splits normally with inspiration. The electrocardiogram reveals right ventricular hypertrophy. A chest x-ray shows dilation of the main pulmonary arteries with decreased vascularity in the outer one-third of the lung fields. The most likely diagnosis is which of the following?

    A. Atrial septal defect
    B. Ventricular septal defect
    C. Congenital pulmonic stenosis
    D. Tetralogy of Fallot
    E. Primary pulmonary hypertension

(See **Medicine: PreTest® Self-Assessment and Review**, 4th ed., #185, answer p. 111.)

In order to answer this question, you don't need to be able to interpret all of the physical findings in this patient. You only need to pay attention to the history. The second and third sentences inform you that she has no history of rheumatic fever or heart murmur and that she was in excellent health until 6 months ago. This information should lead you to eliminate the congenital heart disorders of A, B, C, and D and select the correct answer: E.

Narrow the options Use information in the stem to help you narrow the options. For example:

> For 2 weeks a 3-year old child has experienced petechiae and bleeding of the gums. On examination, he is pale and his temperature is 39° C. This clinical picture is compatible with:
>
> A. Chronic Lymphocytic Leukemia
> B. Acute Lymphocytic Leukemia
> C. Chronic Myelogenous Leukemia
> D. Acute Myelogenous Leukemia
> E. Infectious Mononucleosis

The notation of "2 weeks" in the question rules out "chronic" conditions, A and C. Almost everyone knows someone who has had mononucleosis and common knowledge should lead one to reason that the age and the symptoms of the patient are inconsistent with this disease. At minimum this question can be narrowed to the options B and D. The correct answer is B.

Options meaning the same thing You should look for options which mean the same thing and rule both (all) out since only one answer can be selected (unless, of course, multiple options are possible).

Which of the following tests is the most sensitive and specific for the diagnoses of primary syphilis?

A. Frei test
B. Microhemagglutination *Treponema pallidum* MHA-TP test
C. Venereal Disease Research Laboratories (VDRL) test
D. Automated reagin test
E. Rapid Plasm reagin (RPR) test

(See **Microbiology: PreTest® Self-Assessment and Review**, 6th ed., #141, p. 63 for a discussion of this question.)

Notice that alternatives D and E are tests for the same thing – reagin. While one test may be more sensitive than the other, they test for the same substance and therefore cannot differ in specificity. Therefore, at the outset both choices should be eliminated. Since alternative B is the most specific test (testing for the presence of the organism itself), it should be selected.

3. Elimination Strategies

Once the rules of deductive reasoning have been exhausted, other strategies can help further narrow the options based on the structure of the question and alternatives. Never use any elimination strategies until you have harnessed all of your deductive reasoning skills (see previous section) and applied all your knowledge.

An elimination strategy should never be used to override or substitute for partial knowledge or "reasonable hunches," only as a last resort.

Always look for an absurd option before applying any elimination strategies. The goal of these strategies is to narrow the options and improve guessing performance (the next section) to slightly above chance. Do not expect to get the right answer every time.

Repeating words To eliminate some alternatives, choose the alternative with the most repeating words/themes across the set of alternatives. In other words, alternatives in which words and/or themes repeat in three of the five alternatives are more likely to be correct than others. The following question is an example:

Which of the following pairs of genera are members of the Zygomycetes class and can be seen on microscopic examination to possess rhizoids?

A. Absidia and Mucor
B. Rhizopus and Mucor
C. Rhizopus and Absidia
D. Cladosporium and Rhizopus
E. Cladosporium and Absidia

(See **Microbiology: PreTest® Self-Assessment and Review**, 6th ed., #329, p.119 for a discussion of this question.)

Notice that Rhizopus appears three times in the alternative set (B, C, and D) as does Absidia (A, C, and E). Mucor and Cladosporium only appear twice. Alternative C should be selected, since both its items are repeated the most frequently across alternatives. Also notice the repetition of the root in the word rhizoids from the question itself and in the term Rhizopus; this can be another clue to the correct answer.

A low level of carbon dioxide labeled with ^{14}C is accidentally released into the atmosphere surrounding industrial workers as they resume work following the lunch hour. Unknowingly, they breathe the contaminated air for 2 hours. Which of the following compounds is labeled?

A. Acetyl CoA
B. About one-half the carbon atoms of some fatty acids
C. About one-third the carbon atoms of manonyl CoA
D. The carboxyl atom of fatty acids
E. All the carbon atoms of fatty acids

(See **Biochemistry: PreTest® Self-Assessment and Review**, 6th ed., #237, p. 110 for a discussion of this question.)

In this question, three of the alternatives refer to some quantity (½, ⅓, all) of carbon atoms (B, C, D). One of these should therefore be selected. Since "fatty acids" also repeats across alternatives, in the absence of any knowledge, you would select alternative B on the basis of repeating words. The correct answer, however, is C. Don't forget that you must apply your knowledge before using elimination strategies; the goal of the elimination strategies is simply to improve your odds in the face of uncertainty.

The first (S1 or Lub) heart sound and the second (S2 or Dup) heart sound originate, respectively, from the

A. Closure of the pulmonary valve followed by closure of the aortic valve
B. Closure of the tricuspid valve followed by closure of the mitral valve
C. Closure of the atrioventricular valves followed by closure of the semilunar valves
D. Closure of the atrioventricular valves followed by opening of the semilunar valves
E. Opening of the atrioventricular valves followed by closure of the atrioventricular valves.

(See **Anatomy: PreTest® Self-Assessment and Review**, 6th ed., #199, p. 93 for a discussion of this question.)

The first heart sound is likely to involve "closure of the atrioventricular valves" since this repeats in three alternatives: B, C, and D. We can further narrow the options by observing that the second heart sound is likely to be a closure of something rather than an opening, since "followed by closure of..." repeats in four of the alternatives; this allows us to rule out D, leaving B and C as possible answers. Finally, since "semilunar valves" is repeated twice as an option for the second heart sound (E and C) and nothing else is repeated, we can select C as an answer. <u>Never</u> select an alternative because it doesn't fit the pattern of alternatives; even in EXCEPT, LEAST, or NOT TRUE questions. (See previous example of EXCEPT question.)

Key words Look for key words or parts of key words from the question stem. They are more likely to appear in the correct alternative than in the incorrect alternatives.

Cholera is a toxicogenic dysenteric disease common in many parts of the world. In treatment of patients who have cholera, the use of a drug that inhibits adenyl cyclase would be expected to

A. Kill the patient immediately
B. Eradicate the organism
C. Increase fluid secretion
D. Reduce intestinal motility
E. Block the action of cholera toxin

(See **Microbiology: PreTest® Self-Assessment and Review**, 6th ed., #153, p. 65 for discussion of this question.)

Note that the words from the question, cholera and toxin, repeat in alternative E which happens to be the correct answer.

Avoid absolutes Alternatives with words such as *always*, *never*, *all*, *every*, etc., are more likely to be False than alternatives that do not contain these absolutes. Therefore do not choose them in questions requiring a True statement but consider them in questions requiring a False statement (EXCEPT, LEAST, NOT TRUE, etc).

A major distinction between the methods for producing classical and instrumental condition is that in instrumental conditioning the reinforcing stimulus is
  A. Always appetitive in nature
  B. Contingent on the behavior to be learned
  C. Invariant
  D. Solely under the control of the experimenter
  E. Unnecessary to produce learning

(See **Behavioral Science: PreTest® Self-Assessment and Review**, 5th ed., #155, p. 69 for discussion of this question.)

Alternatives A and D are not likely to be true statements since both contain absolute qualifiers – *always* and *solely*, respectively. If you know nothing else, the options in this question can be effectively narrowed to B, C, and D. The correct answer is B.

All of the following statements regarding the chemotherapy of cancer are true EXCEPT

  A. 50% of all newly diagnosed cancer patients will be cured of their disease
  B. Chemotherapy is the only treatment that can effectively treat systemic disease
  C. Chemotherapy only kills cancer cells and not normal dividing cells
  D. Chemotherapy possesses numerous side effects, such as nausea, vomiting, and suppression of bone marrow
  E. New agents are cell-cycle specific

(See **Pharmacology: PreTest® Self-Assessment and Review**, 6th ed., #76, p. 42 for a discussion of this question.)

In this EXCEPT question, you are looking for a false statement. Since alternatives B and C both contain the absolute qualifier *only*, it is likely that one of these statements is False. In this case the correct answer is C.

Matching answer and question Choose a general answer to general questions and specific answers to specific questions.

Grammar The correct answer should be grammatically consistent with the question. For example, if the question is in the plural, the answer is likely to be in the plural.

Which of the following provides an example of concomitant hyperplasia and hypertrophy?

    A. Uterine growth during pregnancy
    B. Left ventricular cardiac hypertrophy
    C. Enlargement of skeletal muscle in athletics
    D. Breast enlargement at puberty
    E. Cystic hyperplasia of the endometrium

(See **Pathology: PreTest® Self-Assessment and Review**, 6th ed., #1, answer p. 26.)

The correct answer must illustrate <u>both</u> an increase in cell number (hyperplasia) and cell size (hypertrophy). Two of the five alternatives refer to one of these and not both, and can therefore be eliminated. Specifically, alternative B refers only to hypertrophy and E refers only to hyperplasia. The correct answer is A.

Choose long answers An unusually long answer is more likely to be correct than is a shorter answer. But, choose the longest or most specific answer only as a last resort.

4. Guessing Strategies

If more than one option remains after knowledge, reasoning, and elimination strategies have been applied to their full extent, it is time to apply guessing strategies. Use a system to maximize chance.

If you are unable to eliminate any of the alternatives, just choose **A** every time.

If you have narrowed the options somewhat but are left with several choices, just choose the first in the list.

For example, if you must guess between B, C, and D, select B; if you must select between D and E, select D. It is a waste of time and potentially counterproductive to try to select an answer by looking at the visual pattern of the letters on your score sheet preceding your guesses.

If you experience pair-wise confusion among matching questions and alternatives, choose the same alternative for both.

For example, if you know that questions 98 and 99 match with alternatives B and C, but you can't remember which one goes with which, choose B for both. This will guarantee that you get at least one point. If you try to guess correctly, you could lose both points.

When multiple alternatives are possible (i.e., A and C, A, B, and C, or ALL), select the most inclusive answer.

In other words, rule an alternative **IN** (not out) when guessing. There is a slightly higher probability that the most inclusive answer will be correct.

FOR FLEX and FMGEMS EXAMS ONLY

K-Type Questions These questions will not appear on the USMLE, but will continue to appear on FLEX and FMGEMS exams.

Each K-type question contains four suggested responses of which **one or more** may be correct. The question is answered by choosing A if choices 1, 2, and 3 are correct; B if 1 and 3 are correct; C if 2 and 4 are correct; D if only 4 is correct; and E if all are correct. Approach these questions as follows:

Step 1. Try to ELIMINATE one of the options. If you can eliminate any ONE option (1,2,3 or 4), your guessing probability becomes 50%. Retaining any option as correct leaves guessing probability at only 33%. For example, if 1 or 3 is false then only C (2,4) and D (4) need be considered since all other options include 1 and 3. Similarly, if 2 is false you need only consider B (1,3) and D (4) since A, C, and E include option 2. Lastly, if 4 is false, then options A (1,2,3) and B (1,3) are the only possibilities.

Step 2. If you can't rule an option out (i.e., you really don't know), then rule it in. For example, if you have ruled out option 1 and are trying to decide between C(2,4) and D(4), look at option 2 (4 must be true since it is in both). If you can't decide if 2 is true or false, choose C.

Step 3. If you cannot eliminate any alternatives, choose E (all are correct).

Chapter 9

Some Details of Medicine

An alphabetical listing of commonly need-to-know items of information and how to use them.

HOW TO USE This chapter consists of an alphabetical listing of several thousand words and phrases that constitute many but by no means all the details, facts, structures, and concepts of the basic medical sciences. There are several ways in which this chapter may be of use during your review for the USMLE including the following suggestions:

HOW TO USE THE DETAILS

— Periodically browse through the list and allow the items to trigger your memory.

— Write a three-sentence definition or explanation that demonstrates your understanding (not merely recognition) of each item.

— Classify the items according to the dimension system of the USMLE as described in Chapter 1.

— As you review, place a check next to each item that you have considered and understood.

— Look up any item that you either do not recognize or cannot define or explain. After learning the necessary information, circle it in red.

— Each week or so review the circled items to make sure you remember them.

A GUIDE FOR DEALING WITH DETAILS One very useful way to think about the thousands of details of medicine that you must remember is to construct a brief statement of your understanding of the particular detail. It is especially helpful for your memory if you write it out. Also, try to classify the detail according to the following classification system:

CLASSIFICATION OF THE DETAILS

Anatomical structure
Biological substance
Classification
Diagnostic tests
Disease
Drug
Organisms
Process
Socio-behavioral phenomenon

Anatomical structures, such as liver, mast cells, or reticular activating system, should be described in terms of location in the body, gross anatomical and micro/cellular/molecular structure, function and control, pathophysiology, relationships to other structures, effects of aging, and embryological origin.

In the case of each **biological substance,** examples of which include enzymes, hormones, neurotransmitters, etc., you should try to describe its chemical classification and structure, its biological significance, function, synthesis and degradation, its role in disease states if any, and the control of its function.

Kinds of **classification** include blood types, gram-negative organisms, protein synthesis inhibitors, etc. You should describe these in terms of a basic definition of the class, some examples, and why the classification is useful. Also include any limitations in using such a classification system that may exist.

Diagnostic tests and techniques – such as indirect blood pressure measurement, mental status examination, and radioimmunoassay – should be reviewed for how they are used, specificity, sensitivity, and other similar tests. If performed on patients, describe risks, limitations, and costs.

Describe each **disease** (eg., Crohn's disease) in terms of signs and symptoms, differential diagnosis, incidence, treatment, prognosis, pathophysiology, diagnostic tests, etc.

For **drugs** (eg., propranolol), you should know the class, mechanism of action, contraindications, side effects, pharmacokinetics, and other similar drugs.

Nonhuman **organisms**, (eg., *Hemophilus influenzae*) are often important in medicine. You should be able to classify them, describe their anatomy/structure and life cycle, outline their medical significance and, if they are causative agents in disease, give the mechanism, treatment, pathophysiology, etc.

If you are studying a **process** – such as inflammation, aging, protein synthesis, or control of body temperature – be able to give an overall description, pathophysiology, physiological significance, details of the process, relationships to (dependence on) other processes, effects of drugs on the process, and control mechanisms.

Examples of **socio-behavioral phenomenon** include cognitive developmental stages, HMOs, psychoses, etc. Be able to give a general description, significant details, role in human health and illness, and relationships to other such phenomena.

THE DETAILS OF MEDICINE

A
A band
A delta fibers
abdominal oblique
abducens nerve
abductor digiti
abelson leukemia virus
ABOH blood types
absorptive cell, surface
abstract thought
abuse of analgesics
accommodation reflex
acetabular fossa
acetabulum
acetaminophen
acetazolamide
 (Diamox)
acetic acid, titration
 curve
acetoacetate
acetohexamide
acetyl coenzyme A
acetylcholine (ACh)
acetylcholinesterase
acetysalicylic acid
achalasia
achievement tests
achondroplasia
acid-base balance
acidophils
acidosis
acinar glands
aconitase
acromegaly

acrosomal granules
actin (thin) filaments
acting out
actinomycin
action potential
active transport
acute glomerular
 nephritis
acyclovir
acyl groups
adaptation
Addison's disease
adductor
adductor tubercle
adenoassociated virus
adenohypophysis
adenoid tonsils
adenosine
adenoviruses
adenyl cyclase
ADH
adherens
adipocytes
adipose tissue
adluminal compart-
 ment
adolescence
ADP
adrenal cortex
adrenal medulla
Adrenalin
adrenergic receptor(s)
adrenocorticotrophin

adrenogenital
 syndrome
adult polycystic kidney
adventitia
aerotolerant anaerobes
affective disorders
afferent arteriole
afterdischarge
afterload
agammaglobulinemia
aggression
aging
agranular leukocyte
agraphia
airway resistance
akathisia
AKR virus
alanine transaminase
alar laminae
alar plate
albinism
albuterol
alcaptonuria
alcohol dehydrogenase
alcohol, and birth
 defects
alcoholism
aldehyde
aldolase
aldoses
aldosteronism
alkalemia
alkaline phosphatase
alkalosis

alkylating agents
allantois
alleles
allergic encephalitis
allergies
allograft rejection
allopurinol
"all or none" response
allosteric enzymes
alpha cells
alpha globulins
alpha viruses
alpha-1 receptors
alpha-2 receptors
alpha-methyldopa
alternate-form
  reliability
altruism
alveolar epithelium
alveolar gas tensions
alveolar macrophages
alveolar to arterial
  (A-a) O_2 gradient
alveolus
Alzheimer's disease
amacrine cell
amantadine
ambiguous genitalia
ambulatory care
ameloblast
amelogenesis
  imperfecta
amidinocillin
amino acid metabolism
aminoacyl-tRNA
aminopeptidases
aminophylline
aminotransferases
ammonium ion

amnestic syndrome
amniotic fluid
amobarbital
amoebiasis
amoxapine
amoxicillin
AMP from ATP
amphetamine(s)
amphotericin B
ampicillin
ampulla
amygdala
amyl nitrate
amylase
anabolic steroids
anal stage
anaphase
anaphylaxis
anchoring villus
androgen binding
  protein
androgen-insensitivity
androstenedione
androsterone
anemia
angina pectoris
angiotensin I & II
angiotensinogen
animal behavior
animism
anion gap
ankle jerk
annular ligament
anorexia nervosa
antebrachial vein
anterior chamber of
  eye
anterior hypophysis
anthrax

antiandrogens
antianginal agents
antianxiety drugs
antiarrhythmic drugs
antibacterial agents
anticholinergic drugs
anticipatory mourning
anticoagulants
anticodons
antidepressants
antidiarrheals
antidigoxin antibodies
antidiuresis
antidiuretic hormone
antiemetics
antiepileptic drugs
antiestrogens
antifungal agents
antigen presenting
  cells
antigen transporting
  cells
antihelminthics
antihistamines
anti-inflammatory
  drugs
antimalarial drugs
antimanic drugs
antimetabolites
antimycins
antiparasitic agents
antiparkinsonian drugs
antipsychotic drugs
antipyretics
antisocial personality
antispasmodics
antithrombotics
antithyroid drugs
antitussives

antiviral drugs
antrum
anxiety disorders
aorta pressure-volume
aortic regurgitation
aortic stenosis
aortic valve
aphasia
aplastic anemia
apnea
apocrine sweat glands
apomorphine
apoprotein B
appendix
appetite
approach-approach
approach-avoidance
aprindine
APUD cells
aqueous humor
arachidonic acid
arachnoid granulations
arcuate ligament
areola of breast
arginine
aromatic amino acids
arterioles
artificialism
ascorbic acid
ascospores
asparagine
Aspergillus flavus
Aspergillus fumigatus
aspirin
assaultive thoughts
assessment of affect
asthma
astrocytes
astroglia

atelectasis
atenolol
atherosclerosis
atlantoccipital joint
atlas
ATP
atresia
atrial fibrillation
atrial flutter
atrial septal defect
atrioventricular valve
atrioventricular node
atropine
attachment behaviors
attention deficit
  disorder
atypical somatoform
audition
auditory ossicles
Auerbach's plexus
aura
autoimmune disorders
autonomic ganglion
autonomy
autoregulation
autosomal dominant
autosomal recessive
aversive conditioning
avoidance in illness
avoidance-avoidance
avoidant personality
axolemma
azidothymidine (AZT)
azoospermia
azurophilic granules
azygos vein

B
B cell differentiation
B cell growth factor
Babinski reflex
Bachmann's bundle
Bacillus anthracis
Bacillus cereus
bacitracin
baclofen
bacterial flagella
bacteriophages
Bacteroides fragilis
balance
ball and socket joint
barbiturates
baroreceptor reflex
Barr body
basal body
basal electrical rhythm
basal ganglia
basal lamina
basal metabolic rate
base excess
base pairing
basement membrane
basket cells
basophiles
basophilic myelocyte
bedwetting
behaviorism
belief
Bender Visual Motor
  Gestalt Test
benzocaine
benzodiazepines
beriberi
Bernoulli effect
beta agonists
beta antagonists

beta cell
beta-2 receptors
betamethasone
bethanechol
bicarbonate buffer
bile acid
bile salt synthesis
bilirubin
biliverdin
bioavailability
bioenergetics
biofeedback
biogenic amines
biological markers
biotin
biotransformation
bipolar disorder
bipolar neuron
birth control pills
bisexuality
bivalents
bladder cysts
bladder exstrophy
blastocoele
blastomeres
Blastomyces
blastopore
blindness
blood gas(es)
blood lipoproteins
blood pressure
blood transfusion
blood urea nitrogen
blood-brain barrier
bloody show
Blue Cross/Blue Shield
body cavities
body fluids
Bohr effect

bone canaliculi
bone matrix
bony labyrinth
borderline personality
Bordetella
Borrelia
botulism
boutons
bowel
Bowman's capsule
brachial plexus
brachiocephalic vein
bradycardia
bradykinin
brain microglia
brain sand
brain stem
break bone fever
breast milk
breech position
bregma
bretylium
brief reactive psychosis
broad ligament
bromocriptine
bronchiole
bronchitis
bronchodilation
brown adipose tissue
Brucella
Brunner's glands
brush border
buffer system(s)
bulbourethral glands
bulimia
bulk flow
bundle branch block
bundle of His
Burkitt's lymphoma

bursa of Fabricius
butyrophenones

C
C fibers
caffeine
calciferols
calcification zones
calcitonin
California Achieve-
    ment Tests
calmodulin
calorie
calyces of kidney
camper's fascia
Campylobacter fetus
Campylobacter jejuni
canal of Schlemm
cancer chemotherapy
Candida albicans
candidiases
cannabis
capillaries
capsular matrix
captopril
carbachol
carbamino compounds
carbidopa
carbohydrates
carbon dioxide tension
carbon monoxide
carbonic anhydrase
carboxyhemoglobin
carboxypeptidases
cardiac automaticity
cardiac glycosides
cardiac myocytes
cardiac output
cardiac primordium

carotid artery
carotid body
carotid sinus
carpal tunnel syndrome
cartilage calcification
cartwheel nucleus
castration anxiety
cataracts
catatonic schizophrenia
catechol-O-methyl
  transferase
catholic ethics
cation-exchange
cauda equina
cavernous sinus
cefadroxil
celiac disease
celiac ganglia
cell cycle
cell division
cell membrane
cell wall synthesis
cell-mediated immune
  response
cellulitis
cementum
centriole
centroacinar cells
centromeres
cephalosporins
cerebellar plate
cerebellar rudiment
cerebral blood flow
cerebral cortex
cerebral ventricles
cerebrosides
cerebrospinal fluid
ceruloplasmin
cervical dilation

cervical ganglia
cervical mucus plug
cervix
cesarean section
cheesemaker's lung
chelation therapy
chemoreceptors
chemotherapy
chickenpox
chief cells
Chlamydia
Chlamydoconidia
chloral hydrate
chloramphenicol
chloride shift
chloroform
chloroquine
chlorothiazide
chlorpromazine
chlorpropamide
cholecalciferol
cholecystectomy
cholecystokinin
cholesterol synthesis
choline
choline
  acetyltransferase
cholinergic synapse
chondrocytes
chondroitin sulfate
chorda tympani
chordae tendineae
choriocarcinoma
chorion
chorionic gonadotropin
chorionic plate
chorionic villus
  sampling
choroid plexus

chromaffin cells
chromaffin granules
chromatids
chromophobes
chromosome deletions
chronic obstructive
  pulmonary disease
chylomicrons
chyme
chymotrypsin
chymotrypsinogen
cigarette smoking
ciliary body
ciliary ganglia
ciliary muscles
cimetidine
ciprofloxan
circumflex artery
circumstantiality
circumvallate papillae
citric acid cycle
Cladosporium
classical conditioning
clear cell
clearance
cleft palate
clinical interview
clitoris
cloaca
clonidine
Clostridia
club foot
CO_2-titration curve
coarctation of aorta
coated vesicles
cobalt
cocaine
Coccidioides immitis
coccyx

cochlear nerve
cochlear pouch
codeine
codon
coelomic epithelium
coenzyme A
coenzyme Q
cognitive theory
colchicine
collagen
collateral ganglia
collecting ducts
colloid
colloid oncotic
  pressure
color blindness
Colorado tick fever
colostrum
columnar epithelium
coma
compact bone
complement system
computed tomography
conceptus
conditioned reflexes
conducting airway
conduction
cone cells
confabulation
confidentiality
conflict situations
congenital adrenal
  hyperplasia
congenital anomalies
congenital herpes
congestive heart failure
conidia
conjoint tendons
conjunctiva

conscience
consciousness
constipation
construct validity
content validity
contiunous
  reinforcement
contractile component
conus arteriosus
conus elasticus
conus medullaris
cor pulmonale
corneal epithelium
corneal reflex
corona radiata
coronal plane
coronary blood flow
coronary sinus
corpus albicans
corpus callosum
corpus cavernosum
corpus luteum
corpus spongiosum
corpus striatum
cortical nephron
corticopontine tracts
corticospinal tracts
corticosteroidogenesis
corticosterone
corticotropic cells
corticotropin releasing
  hormone
cortisol
cortisol-binding
  globulin
costal processes
costomediastinal
  recess
coumarin

councilman bodies
countercurrent
  exchange
countercurrent
countertransference
Cowper's glands
cowpox virus
Coxiella burnetii
Coxsackie virus
cranial nerves
cremaster
Cri du chat syndrome
cribriform plate
cricoid cartilage
crista terminalis
criterion-based validity
Crohn's disease
cross-bridges
croup
crown-heel length
cruciate ligament
Cryptococcus
cryptorchidism
cubital fossa
cuboidal epithelium
cupula
curare
Cushing reflex
Cushing's syndrome
Cutaneous sensation
cuticle
cyanide poisoning
cyanosis
cyclic AMP
cyclic nucleotides
cycloheximide
cyclooxygenase
cyclosporin
cysteine

cystic duct
cystic fibrosis
cystitis and polyuria
cytochromes
cytomegalovirus
cytotoxic T cells
cytotrophoblast

D
Dale's principle
dark cells
deafness
death and dying
decarboxylase
decerebrate rigidity
decibel unit
decidual cells
Deerfly fever
defecation
deglutition
dehydration states
dehydroepiandrosterone
delirium
delivery
delta cells
delusions
demeclocycline
   (declomycin)
dementia praecox
dendrodendritic
   synapse
dengue
denial
dense bodies
dense connective tissue
dentate nucleus
dentin
deoxycortisol
deoxyhemoglobin

deoxyribonucleic acid
dependent personality
depolarization
depolarization block
depression
dermatomes
DES
desipramine
desmin
desmolase(s)
desmopressin
desmosomes
detoxification
detrusor muscle
deuterium oxide
dexamethasone
dextroamphetamine
dextromethorphan
diabetes insipidus
diabetes mellitus
diabetic ketoacidosis
Diagnostic and Statisti-
   cal Manual of Mental
   Disorders
diagnostic ultrasound
diapedesis
diaphragm
diarrhea
diastasis
diazepam
dicumarol
diencephalon
diethylstilbestrol
differentiation
DiGeorge syndrome
digestion
digestive enzymes
digitalis
digitoxin

digits
diiodotyrosine
dilator muscles
dimers
diopter unit
dipeptidases
diphenylhydantoin
diphtheria
diploidy
dipole
disaccharides
disinfection
displacement behavior
dissociation constant
distal convoluted
   tubule
disulfide bonds
diuretics
dizygotic twins
DNA polymerases
DNA viruses
dominant genes
dopa
dopa decarboxylase
dopamine
dopamine hydroxylase
dorsal horns
dorsal raph nuclei
dorsal root ganglion
dose-response curves
double helix
Down syndrome
DPT vaccine
droperidol
drug-induced lupus
ductus arteriosus
ductus deferens
ductus venosus
duodenal ulcer

dura mater
dust cells
dwarfism
dystonia
dysuria

E
ear
ear rudiments
eating disorders
eccrine sweat glands
echovirus
ectoderm
ectopic kidney
ectopic pregnancy
ED50
edema
Edinger-Westphal
   nucleus
edrophonium
EDTA
effective filtration
   pressure
efferent arteriole
efferent neurons
ego,
ego-ideal
Einthoven's triangle'
ejaculatory duct
elastase
elastic artery
elastic recoil
elastin
electrical synapses
electrical zero
electro-olfactogram
electrocardiogram
electrochemical
   gradient

electroencephalogram
electrolyte composi
   tion
electron transport
   chain
Embden-Meyerhof
   pathway
embryo at 5 weeks
embryoblast
emetics
emetine
empathy
emphysema
empirical validity
emulsification
enamel epithelium
end-plate potential
endocarditis
endocrine glands
endocrinopathies
endolymphatic sac
endonucleases
endopeptidases
endoplasmic reticulum
endorphins
endospores
endotoxins
enkephalins
enolase
enteric fever
enteric nervous system
enterochromaffin cells
enterocolitis
enterotoxin
enteroviruses
enuresis
eosinophilic myelocyte
ependymal layer
ephedrine

epicardium
epididymis
epiglottis
epilepsy
epimers
epinephrine
epiphyseal plate
Epstein-Barr virus
equatorial plate
equilibrium constant
equine encephalitis
   virus
ergocalciferol
ergotamine
Erikson, Erik
erythroblastosis fetalis
erythromycin
erythropoiesis
erythropoietin
Escherichia coli
esophageal atresia
esophageal reflux
essential amino acids
essential fatty acids
estradiol
estriol
estrone
ethacrynic acid
ethanol
ether
ethical relativism
ethmoid bone
ethyl ether
ethylene glycol
eubacterium
eukaryotic cells
excitation-contraction
   coupling

excitatory postsynaptic potential
exocrine gland
exonucleases
exopeptidases
Exophiala werneckii
exophthalmia
exotoxins
expectorants
extended family
extracellular fluid
extracellular matrix
extraembryonic membranes
extrafusal muscle fiber
extrapyramidal system
extravasated urine
eye rudiments
eyetracking dysfunction

F
F-actin
fabricius bursa
face validity
facilitated diffusion
Factor VIII
facultative anaerobes
FADH
Fahraeus-Lindqvist effect
false labor
fascia adherens
fascicle
fasting
fatty acid oxidation
feedback control
female pronucleus
femoral triangle

fenestrated capillaries
fertility drugs
fertilization
fetal alcohol syndrome
fetal circulation
fetal hemoglobin
fibrillation
fibrin
fibrinogen
fibrinolysis
fibroblasts
fibronectin
fibrous astrocyte
Fick principle
Fick's law
fight-or-flight reaction
fila olfactoria
filtered load
filtration fraction
fimbria
first pharyngeal membrane
first pharyngeal pouch
Fischer projections
fixed-ratio reinforcement
flagellum
flat bones
flutter
folic acid
follicle stimulating hormone
follicle-stimulating hormone releasing hormone
food poisoning
foramen of Monro
foramen ovale

forced expiratory volume
fovea centralis
Francisella tularensis
Frank-Starling effect
free energy
free-water clearance
Freud, Sigmund
Friend leukemia virus
frontal plane
fructose 6-phosphate
FSH
fumarate
functional residual capacity
fundic stomach
fungi
furosemide
Fusobacterium

G
G-actin
galactosemia
gallop rhythm
gallstones
galvanometer
gametogenesis
gamma loop
gamma-aminobutyric acid
ganglion layer of retina
gangliosides
gap junctions
gas exchange
gastric secretion
gastric ulcer
gastrin
gastrulation
Gaucher's disease

gender identity
general anesthetics
generalized anxiety
generator potential
genetic code
genetic manipulation
geniculate ganglia
genome
germ layers
German measles
germinal epithelium
gestational age
giant pyramidal cells
giantism
glaucoma
glial cells
glomerular filtration
   rate
glomerulus
glossopharyngeal
   nerve
glucagon
glucocorticoids
glucokinase
gluconeogenesis
glucose 6-phosphatase
glucostatic theory
glucuronic acid
glutamine
glutathione
gluten
gluteus maximus
glycerol
glycerol kinase
glycerol phosphate
   shuttle
glycine
glycocalyx
glycogen

glycogen synthetase
glycogenolysis
glycolysis
glycoproteins
glycosides
goblet cells
goiter
Golgi apparatus
Golgi neurons
gonadal agenesis
gonadal dysgenesis
gonadotropes
gonadotropin releasing
   hormone
gonadotropins
gonococcal infections
Goodpasture's
   syndrome
gout
Graafian follicle
gracilis
graft-versus-host
granulosa cells
grasp reflex
Graves' disease
gray baby syndrome
gray matter
greater omentum
grief
griseofulvin
group behavior
growth hormone
guanosine triphosphate
Guillain-Barre
   syndrome
guilt feelings
gum
gustatory
gynecoid pelvis

gynecomastia

H
H band
H-1 receptors
H-2 receptors
habituation
hair bulb
hair cells,
Haldane effect
half-life of drugs
hallucinations
hallucinogens
haloperidol
halothane
haploid pronuclei
Hartnup's disease
Haversian canal
hay fever
hemoglobin F
heart block
heart murmur
heart rate
heavy meromyosin
heavy metal poisoning
helicotrema
helix
helper T cells
hematopoiesis
heme
hemodynamics
hemoglobin
hemoglobinopathies
hemolytic anemia
Hemophilus
hemopoietic tissue
hemosiderin
hemostatic agents
hemothorax

Henderson-Hasselbach
equation
Henle's loop
Henry's law
heparin
hepatic acinus
hepatic duct
hepatic vein
hepatitis B
hepatomegaly
herbicides
hernia
heroin
Herpes simplex
Herring bodies
heterozygotes
hexamethonium
hexokinase
high density lipopro-
teins
hip dysplasia
hippocampus
Hippocratic tradition
hirsutism
histamine
histocompatibility
antigens
histones
*Histoplasma
capsulatum*
HIV infection
holocrine gland
homeostasis
homocysteine
homosexuality
homozygotes
Hook's law
hormone-sensitive
lipase

Horner's syndrome
human adenoviruses
human chorionic
gonadotropin
human leukocyte
antigens
human placental
lactogen
human T-cell leukemia
viruses
hunger
Huntington's disease
hyalurinidases
hydatidiform mole
hydralazine
hydrocephalus
hydrochlorothiazide
hydrogen bonds
hymen
hyoid arch
hyperaldosteronism
hypercalcemia
hypercapnia
hyperglycemia
hyperkalemia
hyperkeratinization
hyperlipidemia
hyperosmolality
hyperphosphaturia
hyperpnea
hyperprolactinemia
hypertension
hyperthermia
hyperthyroidism
hyperventilation
hypnotics
hypogastric nerve
hypoglycemia
hypokalemia

hypophyseal portal
system
hypotension
hypothalamohypophyseal
tract
hypothalamus
hypothyroidism
hypoventilation and
hypoxia
hypovolemia
hypoxia

I
I bands
ibuprofen
id
iliac crest
ilium
illusions
image formation
imipramine
immune response
immunoassays
immunoelectrophoresis
immunoglobulins
impetigo
implantation
impotence
imprinting
in vitro fertilization
incisura
inclusion bodies
incus
individuation
indomethacin
inferior colliculus
inferior vena cava
infertility
influenza viruses

lactogenic hormone
lactose (lac) operon
lactose intolerance
lamellae
lamina propria
larynx
lateral geniculate
  nucleus
lateral inhibition
lateral ventricles
law of electroneutrality
law of Laplace
laxatives
lean body mass
learned helplessness
learning
Legionella
pneumophila
leishmaniasis
length-tension
  relationship
lens
leprosy
Leptospiro
lethal dose,mean
  (LD50)
leucine
leukotriene synthesis
levodopa
Leydig (interstitial)
  cells
LH
libido
licensing of physicians
lidocaine
ligamentum flavum
light cell
light meromyosin
lincomycin

linea alba
linea aspera
linea terminalis
Lineweaver-Burk
  equation
lingual glands
lingual tonsils
lingula
linolenic acid
lipase
lipid storage cells
lipoproteins
lipotropic hormone
Listeria monocyto-
  genes
lithium
load-volocity
local anesthetics
locus ceruleus
loop diuretics
loop of Henle
lordosis
low density lipopro-
  teins
lumbar puncture
luteinizing hormone
Lyme disease
lymph
lymph nodes
lymphoblast
lymphocyte
lymphokines
lysergic acid
  diethylamide
lysine
lysosome
lysozyme

M
M cell
M line in H band
macrophages
macula densa cells
magnesium sulfate
magnetic resonance
  imaging
major histocompatibil-
  ity complex
Malassezia furfur
malate
malignant
  hyperthermia
malingering
malleus
mammary glands
mania
mannitol
MAO inhibitors
Maple syrup urine
  disease
Marburg virus
Marfan's syndrome
marijuana
mast cells
mastoid processus
maximal voluntary
  ventilation
measles virus
mechanoreceptors
meclofenamate
median eminence
mediastinum
Medicaid
medical malpractice
Medicare
megakaryoblast
meiosis

Meissner's corpuscle
Meissner's plexus
melanocyte
melanocyte-
  stimulating hormone
melatonin
membrane potential
membranous labyrinth
memory B cells
memory T cells
menarche
meningitis
menopause
menstrual cycle
meprobamate
Merkel cells
merocrine glands
mescaline
mesenchymal cells
messenger RNA
met-enkephalin
metabolic acidosis
metabolic alkalosis
metanephrine
metanephros
metaphase
metarteriole
metastasis
metazoan infections
methadone
methamphetamine
methanol
methemoglobinemia
methionine
methotrexate
methylcellulose
methyldopa
methylxanthines
micelles

Michaelis-Menten
  equation
microencephaly
microfilament
microgli
Microsporum
microtubule
microvilli
micturition
middle ear ossicle
midlife crisis
migraine
milk ejection reflex
mineralocorticoids
miniature end-plate
  potential
Minnesota Multiphasic
  Personality Inventory
mitochondria
mitosis
mitral valve
monoamine oxidase
monoaminergic
  neurons
monozygotic twins
mood disorders
morphine
motor end plate
mucin
mucopolysaccharides
mucous neck cells
multifactorial
  inheritance
multiple sclerosis
multipolar neuron
mumps virus
muscarinic
  cholinoceptors
muscle contraction

muscle twitch
mutations
myasthenia gravis
Mycobacteria
Mycoplasma
mycoses
mydriasis
myelin sheath
myenteric plexus
myoblasts
myocardial infarction
myoepithelial cells
myofibrils
myoglobin
myometrium
myoneural junction
myosin filaments
myxedema

N
NADH
NADP
nails
narcolepsy
nasal placodes
nasolacrimal duct
nasopharynx
neclear chain muscle
  fiber
negative feedback
Neisseria
nematode infections
neologisms
neomycin
neonate
neostigmine
nephrotoxicity
Nernst equation
nerve impulse

neural crest cells
neural groove
neural tube
neuraminidase
neuroblasts
neuroectoderm
neuroendocrine
neurofilament
neuroglia
neurohypophysis
neuroleptics
neuromodulators
neurosecretion
neurotensin
neurotransmitter
neutrophil
niacin
nicotinamide
nicotine
nigrostriatal tract
Nissl bodies
nitrates
nitrites
nitrogen washout test
nitrogen balance
nitrogen mustards
nitroglycerin
nitrous oxide
nociceptors
node of Ranvier
non-REM sleep
norepinephrine
norethindrone
normetanephrine
notochord
nuclear bag fibers
nuclear chain fibers
nuclear family
nucleic acids

nucleolus
nucleotides
nutrient transport
nystatin

O
obesity
object permanence
obligate aerobes
obligate anaerobes
obsessions
obstetrics
occipital sinus
oculomotor nerve
odor discrimination
oedipal stage
Ohm's law
olfactory bulb
olfactory epithelium
olfactory hallucina-
    tions
olfactory nerve
oligodendroglia
oligosaccharides
oligospermia
olivary nucleus
oncogenes
oogenesis
oogonia
operant conditioning
operons
opiates
opioid peptides
Opthalmia neonatorum
optic chiasm
optic disc
oral contraceptives
organ of Corti
osmolar gap

osmotic agents
osmotic diuresis
ossicles
ossification
osteoblast
osteoclast
otic vesicle
otolith
ototoxicity
outer fiber, rod cell
oval window
ovarian follicle
oxaloacetate
oxygen dissociation
    curve
oxyntic cells
oxytocin
ozone

P
pacemaker cells
Pacinian corpuscle
pain
palmitate
palsy
pancreaozymin
pancreatic acinar cells
pancreatic buds
pancreatic islet
pancreatic polypeptide
pancrelipase
panic disorder
papaverine
papillary muscles
para-aminohippuric
    acid
Paracoccidioides
paracrine cells
parallel play

potency
poxviruses
PPD test
preanesthetic drugs
precapillary sphincter
prednisone
pregnancy
pregnenalone
pressure pulse
pressure-volume
  curves
presynaptic inhibition
presynaptic membrane
primary bronchi
primary follicle
primitive streak
probenecid
procaine
procarbazine
procollagen
progesterone
progestins
prognathism
prohormone
prokaryotic cells
prolactin
promethazine
promoter
pronephros
prophase
propranolol
propylthiouracil
prostacyclins
prostaglandin(s)
protein hormones
protestant ethics
prothrombin
protodiastole
proton pump

protoporphyrin IX
proximal convoluted
  tubule
pseudocholinesterase
Pseudomonas
psilocybin
psoas
psychoanalysis
psychogenic pain
psychosis
psyllium
ptyalin
puberty
pubic crest
public health
pulmonary complaince
pulmonary emboli
pulmonary function
  tests
pulse
purkinje cells
puromycin
pyloric glands
pylorus
pyramidal cells
pyrimidines
pyrloric stenosis
pyruvate kinase

Q
Q fever
quadriceps femoris
quadruplets
quaternary structure
quickening
quinidine syncope
quinine

R
rabbit fever
rabies virus
radial nerve
radioimmunoassay
radius
rami communicantes
raphe nuclei
Rathke's pouch
reaction formation
recombinant DNA
red muscle fiber
red nucleus
reflex arc
refractive power
refractory period
regression
reinforcement
relaxin
releasing hormones
reliability of tests
religious ethics
REM sleep
renal blood flow
renal calyx
renal plasma flow
renin-angiotensin
rennin
reoviruses
repair of DNA
replication of DNA
repression
reserpine
respiratory acidosis
respiratory alkalosis
respiratory control
respiratory quotient
resting membrane
  potential

rete testis
reticular activating
    system
reticular formation
reticulocyte
retroviruses
reversal potential
reverse transcriptase
Reye's syndrome
Reynold's number
Rh antigens
rheumatic fever
rheumatoid arthritis
rhinitis
Rhizopus
rhodopsin
rhombencephalon
riboflavin
ribonucleic acid
ribose 5-phosphate
ribosomal RNA
Rickettsia
right axis deviation
right subclavian artery
right ventricular
    hypertrophy
ringworm
RNA polymerase
RNA viruses
rod cells
Roman Catholic ethics
Rorschach Inkblot Test
rostral
rotator cuff
rotaviruses
rotenone
rough endoplasmic
    reticulum
round window

rubella virus
Ruffini's corpuscles
rule-based ethics
rules of logic

S
S-1 receptors
S-2 receptors
sagittal sinus
sagittal suture
salicylate(s)
saliva
salivary amylase
Salmonella
saltatory conduction
Sandfly fever virus
saphenous nerve
saphenous vein
sarcolemma
sarcomere
sarcoplasmic reticulum
scala vestibuli
scapular notch
Scarlet fever
Schiff's base
schizophrenia
Schlemm canal
Schwann cells
sciatic nerve
sclerotome
scoliosis
scopolamine
seasonal affective
    disorder
sebaceous glands
secobarbital
second messengers
secondary structure
secretin

secretory granules
sedati
seizure
self-determination
sella turcica
semen
semicircular canal
semilunar valve
septicemia
series elastic
    component
serotonin
serous glands
Sertoli cells
serum proteins
serum sickness
sexual dimorphism
Shigella
shock
sick sinus syndrome
sickle cell anemia
sigmoid colon
signal sequence
simple diffusion
simple epithelium
single-gene defects
sinoatrial node
sinus venosus
sinusoids
Skinner, B.F.
sleep states
slow calcium channel
slow viruses
smoking
smooth muscle
social drugs
sodium-hydrogen
    pump

sodium-potassium pump
solubility constant (s)
solvent drag
soma
somatomedins
somatostatin
somatotropic cell
somatotropi
somites
sound waves
Southern blotting
space constant
Space of Disse
spasticity
spatial summation
spermatogenesis
sphingolipids
sphingomyelin
spina bifida
spinal shock
spiral ganglion
spirochetes
spironolactone
splanchnic mesoderm
splanchnic nerve
splicing of RNA
spongy bone
sprue
squamous epithelium
St. Louis encephalitis virus
Stanford-Binet scale
stapedius
Staphylococcus aureus
Starling effect
startle reflex
starvation
steady stat

steatorrhea
stereocilia
stereoisomers
sternohyoid
steroid metabolism
stimulants
stomodeum
stratified epithelium
Streptococci
streptokinase
streptomycin
stress
stroke volume
subarachnoid hemorrhage
subclavian vein
subdural hemorrhage
sublingual glands
submandibular glands
substance abuse
substantia nigra
succinyl CoA
succinylcholine
succus entericus
sucking reflex
suicidal thoughts
sulcus terminalis
sulfadoxine
sulfamethoxazole
sulfhydryl group
sulfisoxazole
sulfonamides
sulfonylurea(s)
summation
superior colliculus
superior vena cava
superoxide dismutase
suppression
suppressor T cells

supraoptic nucleus
surfactant
SV-40 virus
sweat glands
sympathetic ganglia
sympathomimetic drugs
symphysis pubis
synaptic cleft
synaptic membrane
synaptic transmission
syncope
syncytial giant cells
syncytium
synovial fluid
syphilis
systematic desensitization
systole

T
T tubule
tachycardia
tachypnea
tail bud
tanycyte
tardive dyskinesia
taste bud
Tay-Sachs disease
TCA cycle
tear
tegmentum
tela choroidea
telencephalon
telophase
temporal fossa
teniae coli
terminal bronchiole
terminal web

terpin hydrate
terrible twos
tertiary structure
testosterone
tetanus
tetracycline(s)
tetraiodothyronine
Tetralogy of Fallot
tetraploidy
thalamus
thalassemia
thalidomide
theca externa
theca folliculi
theca interna
theophylline
therapeutic index
thiazide diuretics
thick myofilament
thin myofilament
thin segment
thiocyanate
thiolase
thiopental
thoracic duct
threonine
threshold potential
thrombolytics
thromboxanes
thrush
thyroglobulin
thyroid follicle
thyrosine
thyrotropic cells
thyroxine (T4)
tibial condyles
tight junctions
time constant
timolol

Tinea
tissue plasminogen
titratable acid
tobacco use
tolazamide
tolazoline
tolbutamide
tongue papilla
tooth bud
total body water
total lung capacity
Tourette syndrome
toxic shock syndrome
toxicology
toxoplasma
trabeculae
tranquilizers
transcription
transduction
transfer RNA
transference
translocation
transmural pressures
transpeptidases
trematode infections
Treponema pallidum
triad
tricarboxylic acid cycle
triceps brachii
Trichophyton
Trichosporon
tricuspid atresia
tricyclic antidepres-
  sants
trigeminal neuralgia
triglycerides
triiodothyronine (T3)
trilaminar gastrula
tripeptidases

triploidy
tRNA
trochlear nerve
trophic hormone
trophoblast
tropomyosin
troponin complex
true ribs
truncus arteriosus
trypsinogen
tryptophan
tubal pregnancy
tuber cinereum
tuberculosis
Tuberculum
tubocurarine
tubulin
tularemia
tumor necrosis factor
tumor viruses
Turner syndrome
tympanic membrane
tyrosine hydroxylase

U
ubiquinone
UDP-galactose
UDP-glucose
ulcerative colitis
ulnar bursae
ultimobranchial bodies
ultrasonography
umbilical artery
unipolar disorder
unipolar neuron
unit membrane
uracil mustard
urea cycle
Ureaplasma

urealyticum
ureteric bud
urethra
uricosuric agents
urogenital folds
urokinase
utilitarianism
utricle
uvea
uvula

V
vaccines
Vaccinia virus
vagus nerve
valine
Valley fever
valsalva maneuver
values
van't Hoff equation
vancomycin
vanillylmandelic acid
variola
vas deferens
vasa recta
vasa vasorum
vascular resistance
vasoconstriction
vasodilation
vasomotion
vasopressin
velocity of flow
vena cava
venoconstriction
venous return
ventilation:perfusion
    ratio
ventricular fibrillation
ventricular arrhythmias

verapamil
vertebral arches
very low-density
    lipoprotein
vestibular apparatus
Vibrio
vibrissae
villi
vinblastine
viral capsid
viral genome
viral infections
vision
visual purple
vital capacity
vitamins
voltage gated channels
volume of distribution
vulva

W
warfarin
Wechsler Intelligence
    Tests
white adipose tissue
white blood cell
white muscle fiber
whooping cough
wild-type allele
Witch's milk
Wolffian ducts

X
X chromosome
xanthine oxidase
xiphoid processus
XO genotype
XXX genotype
XXY genotype

xylulose 5-phosphate
XYY genotype

Y
Y chromosome
yaws
yeast infections
yellow bone marrow
yellow fever
Yersinia
yolk sac

Z
Z line
Zollinger-Ellison
    syndrome
zona fasciculata
zona glomerulosa
zona pellucida
zona reticularis
zygomatic arch
zygomatic nerve
zygote
zymogen granules
zymogenic cells

Chapter 10

A Final Word

Something for you to think about a few days before you take your USMLE.

When you have conscientiously applied the information, tips, and suggestions offered in this book, you should be well prepared to take the USMLE. This thought, "I am well prepared," will help you relax and give you confidence in yourself as the test date approaches.

On the day before the examination, we recommend that you choose a time to stop studying (3 or 4 in the afternoon), and then really stop. A few more hours so close to the exam will make little difference to your score. Close your books, put away your notes and charts, and congratulate yourself on a job well done.

If you adhered to your review plan, spend the remainder of the evening enjoying a relaxing dinner, and, hopefully, a good night's sleep.

As you enter the test site, remember: **You are well prepared**. Your planning and hard work can give you the confidence and concentration to apply all that you have learned to do well on the exam.

We hope that your experience with the USMLE is successful and as pleasant as possible. If you carefully planned and reviewed, you should do well on the test.

We hope this book helped you do that.

STUDY SUGGESTION

Summarizing and reorganizing information by making charts, drawing pictures or diagrams, and mentally visualizing are all active learning strategies that promote long-term retention.

CONSIDERATION OF THE QUESTION ON PAGE 162

Decision #1 - Does this disease involve epinephrine (mentioned twice), cortisol (mentioned twice), or vasopression (mentioned once)? The adrenal cortex synthesizes cortisol, and the adrenal medulla synthesizes epinephrine, vasopression is associated with the pituitary. Alternatives D and E are the only viable options.

Decision #2 - Would there be an increase (D) or a decrease in the production of cortisol (E) with this disease? Cushing's disease involves an overproduction of cortisol, hence the correct answer is D. Notice that "excessive" repeats in three alternatives.

APPENDIX
ANSWERS TO PRACTICE TESTS

ANATOMY-I

1 C Embryology
2 D Embryology
3 B Histology
4 E Neuroanatomy
5 A Head & Neck
6 E Histology
7 E Histology
8 B Thorax
9 B Thorax
10 C Abdomen
11 B Pelvis
12 E Thorax
13 C Abdomen
14 C Abdomen
15 B Neuroanatomy
16 B Neuroanatomy
17 A Pelvis
18 B Pelvis
19 A Head & Neck
20 C Extremities & Back
21 E Neuroanatomy
22 C Head & Neck
23 D Extremities & Back
24 A Histology
25 C Head & Neck

ANATOMY-II

1 A Embryology
2 B Embryology
3 C Histology
4 B Histology
5 D Histology
6 B Histology
7 A Histology
8 C Thorax
9 A Abdomen
10 D Pelvis
11 C Abdomen
12 D Pelvis
13 E Head and Neck
14 A Head and Neck
15 C Thorax
16 B Extremities & Back
17 C Head and Neck
18 C Extremities & Back
19 A Extremities & Back
20 A Neuroanatomy
21 D Neuroanatomy
22 B Neuroanatomy
23 C Neuroanatomy
24 D Pelvis
25 B Extremities & Back

BEHAVIOR-I

1 C Biological Correlates
2 C Biological Correlates
3 E Biological Correlates
4 E Biological Correlates
5 C Behavioral Genetics
6 C Behavioral Genetics
7 D Behavior&Personality
8 D Behavior&Personality
9 C Development
10 A Family,Community
11 D Development
12 C Communication
13 C Communication
14 E Group Processes
15 E Learning & Behavior
16 B Group Processes
17 D Family,Community
18 B Sociocultural
19 B Sociocultural
20 D Disease
21 D Disease
22 D Risk Factors
23 D Risk Factors
24 B Health Care
25 E Statistics & Design

BEHAVIOR–II

1 D Biological Correlates
2 C Biological Correlates
3 C Biological Correlates
4 C Behavioral Genetics
5 B Behavioral Genetics
6 C Behavior&Personality
7 D Behavior&Personality
8 B Learning & Behavior
9 D Learning & Behavior
10 A Development
11 B Sociocultural
12 A Development
13 B Communication
14 A Health Care
15 C Group Processes
16 C Group Processes
17 C Disease
18 A Family, Community
19 D Sociocultural
20 D Risk Factors
21 E Disease
22 E Risk Factors
23 A Health Care
24 A Statistics & Design
25 E Statistics & Design

BIOCHEMISTRY–I

1 C Amino Acids, Proteins, &Enzymes
2 A Amino Acids, Proteins, &Enzymes
3 B Amino Acids, Proteins, &Enzymes
4 A Nucleic Acids
5 D Amino Acids, Proteins, &Enzymes
6 C Amino Acids, Proteins, &Enzymes
7 E Nucleic Acids
8 C Nucleic Acids
9 D Nucleic Acids
10 A Nucleic Acids
11 B Nucleic Acids
12 D Carbohydrates and Lipids
13 A Carbohydrates and Lipids
14 B Carbohydrates and Lipids
15 D Vitamins and Hormones
16 E Vitamins and Hormones
17 D Vitamins and Hormones
18 E Vitamins and Hormones
19 B Membranes and Cell Structure
20 C Metabolism
21 C Metabolism
22 D Metabolism
23 A Metabolism
24 B Amino Acids, Proteins & Enzymes
25 A Amino Acids, Proteins & Enzymes

BIOCHEMISTRY–II

1 B Amino Acids, Proteins & Enzymes
2 A Amino Acids, Proteins & Enzymes
3 D Amino Acids, Proteins & Enzymes
4 A Amino Acids, Proteins & Enzymes
5 B Vitamins and Hormones
6 D Amino Acids, Proteins & Enzymes
7 E Nucleic Acids
8 D Nucleic Acids
9 B Carbohydrates and Lipids
10 C Nucleic Acids
11 C Nucleic Acids
12 B Carbohydrates and Lipids
13 C Carbohydrates and Lipids
14 A Nucleic Acids
15 A Carbohydrates and Lipids
16 C Vitamins and Hormones
17 B Vitamins and Hormones
18 C Metabolism
19 C Membranes and Cell Structure
20 D Membranes and Cell Structure
21 E Membranes and Cell Structure
22 A Carbohydrates and Lipids
23 C Metabolism
24 D Metabolism
25 C Metabolism

GENETICS

1	A
2	B
3	C
4	B
5	B
6	D
7	C
8	D
9	D
10	D
11	B
12	E

13	A
14	B
15	C
16	D
17	B
18	D
19	C
20	A
21	B
22	B
23	A
24	C
25	D

MICROBIOLOGY–I

1	B	Virology
2	D	Virology
3	A	Virology
4	D	Immunology
5	E	Virology
6	B	Bacteriology
7	E	Bacteriology
8	D	Bacteriology
9	C	Bacteriology
10	C	Bacteriology
11	E	Physiology
12	C	Physiology
13	D	Immunology

14	A	Rickettsiae, Chlamydiae, & Mycoplasmas
15	D	Rickettsiae, Chlamydiae, & Mycoplasmas
16	C	Mycology
17	B	Mycology
18	E	Parasitology
19	D	Immunology
20	C	Immunology
21	D	Physiology
22	E	Mycology
23	D	Virology
24	C	Rickettsiae, Chlamydiae, & Mycoplasmas
25	C	Parasitology

MICROBIOLOGY–II

1	B	Virology
2	C	Bacteriology
3	B	Virology
4	D	Immunology
5	A	Bacteriology
6	C	Virology
7	A	Bacteriology
8	A	Bacteriology
9	D	Virology
10	A	Immunology
11	D	Physiology
12	C	Physiology
13	E	Mycology

14	C	Mycology
15	D	Rickettsiae, Chlamydiae and Mycoplasmas
16	B	Rickettsiae, Chlamydiae and Mycoplasmas
17	A	Mycology
18	D	Physiology
19	B	Parasitology
20	C	Bacteriology
21	C	Immunology
22	A	Parasitology
23	E	Virology
24	D	Parasitology
25	C	Immunology

NEUROSCIENCE

1 C Neuron Functions
2 A Neuron Functions
3 C Neuron Functions
4 A Neuron Functions
5 C Motor
6 C Higher Functions
7 H or G Transmitters
8 E Transmitters
9 D Transmitters
10 A Transmitters
11 D Transmitters
12 B Spinal Cord
13 C Spinal Cord
14 A Sensory
15 B Spinal Cord
16 A Brainstem and Cranial Nerves
17 A Brainstem and Cranial Nerves
18 E Brainstem and Cranial Nerves
19 F Brainstem and Cranial Nerves
20 E Brainstem and Cranial Nerves
21 E Sensory
22 C Sensory
23 D Motor
24 B Higher Functions
25 A Spinal Cord

PATHOLOGY–I

1 B General Pathology
2 D Respiratory System
3 A Genitourinary System
4 C General Pathology
5 A Cardiovascular System
6 B Hematology
7 E Cardiovascular System
8 C Respiratory System
9 D Gastrointestinal System
10 D Respiratory System
11 D Gastrointestinal System
12 E Genitourinary System
13 C Genitourinary System
14 B Nervous System
15 C General Pathology
16 C Musculoskeletal System
17 A General Pathology
18 B Nervous System
19 A Genitourinary System
20 C Musculoskeletal System
21 B Nervous System
22 A General Pathology
23 C Endocrine System
24 C Skin & Breast
25 B Hematology

PATHOLOGY–II

1 A General Pathology
2 D General Pathology
3 C General Pathology
4 C Hematology
5 D Hematology
6 A Hematology
7 B Cardiovascular
8 D Cardiovascular
9 D Respiratory
10 C Respiratory
11 D Gastrointestinal
12 B Respiratory
13 E Gastrointestinal
14 A Gastrointestinal
15 B Genitourinary
16 C Genitourinary
17 C Genitourinary
18 D Nervous System
19 B Endocrine
20 E Nervous System
21 C Musculoskeletal System
22 B Musculoskeletal System
23 E Skin and Breast
24 B Skin and Breast
25 D Nervous System

PHARMACOLOGY–I

1 B General Principles
2 D Chemotherapy
3 C Central Nervous System
4 C Toxicology
5 C Chemotherapy
6 A Chemotherapy
7 B Toxicology
8 D Chemotherapy
9 C Central Nervous System
10 A Cardiovascular System
11 E Renal System
12 C Cardiovascular System
13 D Central Nervous System
14 C Cardiovascular System
15 C Autonomic Nervous System
16 D Central Nervous System
17 D Endocrine System
18 A Chemotherapy
19 B Renal System
20 D Renal System
21 D Endocrine System
22 D Autonomic Nervous System
23 E Endocrine System
24 A General Principles
25 A Chemotherapy

PHARMACOLOGY–II

1 A General Principles
2 C General Principles
3 C Chemotherapy
4 B General Principles
5 A Chemotherapy
6 C Chemotherapy
7 D Central Nervous System
8 C Chemotherapy
9 D Autonomic Nervous System
10 A Toxicology
11 D Toxicology
12 D Central Nervous System
13 C Central Nervous System
14 E Autonomic Nervous System
15 A Autonomic Nervous System
16 B Cardiovascular System
17 C Cardiovascular System
18 D Cardiovascular System
19 B Cardiovascular System
20 D Renal System
21 D Renal System
22 E Renal System
23 D Endocrine System
24 B Endocrine System
25 E Endocrine System

PHYSIOLOGY–I

1 B Metabolism & Endocrinology
2 D Metabolism & Endocrinology
3 D Metabolism & Endocrinology
4 B Metabolism & Endocrinology
5 A Metabolism & Endocrinology
6 B Metabolism & Endocrinology
7 C Cardiovascular System: Vascular
8 D Cardiovascular System: Vascular
9 E Cardiovascular System: Vascular
10 A Cardiovascular System: Heart
11 A Cardiovascular System: Vascular
12 B Cardiovascular System: Vascular
13 A Cardiovascular System: Vascular
14 C Cardiovascular System: Heart
15 B Cardiovascular System: Heart
16 C Respiratory System
17 B Respiratory System
18 E Respiratory System
19 A Respiratory System
20 A Respiratory System
21 B Renal and Acid-Base Physiology
22 C Renal and Acid-Base Physiology
23 B Gastrointestinal System
24 C Gastrointestinal System
25 A Gastrointestinal System

PHYSIOLOGY–II

1 E Metabolsim and Endocrinology
2 A Cardiovascular System: Vascular
3 A Metabolsim and Endocrinology
4 E Gastrointestinal System
5 C Cellular Physiology
6 E Renal and Acid-Base Physiology
7 E Cardiovascular System: Vascular
8 C Gastrointestinal System
9 D Cardiovascular System: Vascular
10 B Cardiovascular System: Heart
11 A Cardiovascular System: Heart
12 B Cardiovascular System: Heart
13 C Respiratory System
14 B Metabolsim and Endocrinology
15 C Respiratory System
16 E Metabolsim and Endocrinology
17 E Renal and Acid-Base Physiology
18 C Renal and Acid-Base Physiology
19 A Gastrointestinal System
20 E Gastrointestinal System
21 C Neurophysiology
22 E Neurophysiology
23 D Neurophysiology
24 D Respiratory System
25 E Cellular Physiology

STUDY SUGGESTION

Your weakest topics should receive more time and effort than your stronger subjects but do not neglect your strongest subjects entirely. There is a law of diminishing returns when it comes to reviewing for the USMLE: the better you know the material, the less you stand to gain by investing a lot of time reviewing. Conversely, the less well you know the material, the more you can gain by study.